# Notes on Anatomy and Oncology

*For Churchill Livingstone:*

*Senior Commissioning Editor:* Sarena Wolfaard
*Project Development Manager:* Dinah Thom
*Project Manager:* Ailsa Laing
*Designer:* Judith Wright

# Notes on Anatomy and Oncology

**David O'Halloran** BEd(Hons) MEd DHSM DCR(T) ILTM
Director, O'Halloran Consultancy Limited; Accreditor for the
Institute for Learning and Teaching in Higher Education; Formerly
Senior Lecturer in Radiotherapy, School of Healthcare Studies,
University of Leeds, Leeds, UK

**Kathryn Guyers** BSc DCR(T) CTCert
Lecturer in Radiotherapy, School of Healthcare Studies,
University of Leeds, Leeds, UK

**Jill Henderson** BHSc(Hons) PGCE DCR(T)
Lecturer in Radiotherapy, School of Healthcare Studies,
University of Leeds, Leeds, UK

Foreword by

**April G Fritz** BA RHIT CTR
Registered Health Information Technician and Tumor Registrar,
Gaithersburg MA, USA

*Illustrations by Graeme Chambers BA(Hons)*
*Medical Artist*

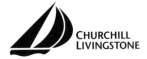

CHURCHILL
LIVINGSTONE

EDINBURGH  LONDON  NEW YORK  OXFORD  PHILADELPHIA  ST LOUIS  SYDNEY  TORONTO  2004

CHURCHILL LIVINGSTONE
An imprint of Elsevier Limited

First published 2004
  Reprinted 2005, 2006

ISBN 0 443 07322 8

British Library Cataloguing in Publication Data
A catalogue record for this book is available from the British Library

Library of Congress Cataloguing in Publication Data
A catalogue record for this book is available from the Library of Congress

Note
Medical knowledge is constantly changing. Standard safety precautions must be followed, but as new research and clinical experience broaden our knowledge, changes in treatment and drug therapy may become necessary or appropriate. Readers are advised to check the most current product information provided by the manufacturer of each drug to be administered to verify the recommended dose, the method and duration of administration, and contraindications. It is the responsibility of the practitioner, relying on experience and knowledge of the patient, to determine dosages and the best treatment for each individual patient. Neither the Publisher nor the author assumes any liability for any injury and/or damage to persons or property arising from this publication.

The Publisher

ELSEVIER   your source for books,
           journals and multimedia
           in the health sciences
**www.elsevierhealth.com**

Working together to grow
libraries in developing countries

www.elsevier.com | www.bookaid.org | www.sabre.org

ELSEVIER   BOOK AID   Sabre Foundation
           International

The
publisher's
policy is to use
paper manufactured
from sustainable forests

Printed in China

# Contents

# Foreword

The English and Americans are two peoples separated by a common language.

This famous phrase has been variously attributed to Oscar Wilde, George Bernard Shaw, Winston Churchill, Bertrand Russell, and even to John Cleese of Monty Python fame. There is considerable truth to the phrase, even beyond the obvious spelling differences between the two versions of the language. However, even more acutely felt than the differences between the English and Americans are language and terminology differences within each culture—especially between physicians and cancer data collectors.

The people who collect cancer information on individual patients—variously called abstractors, tumor registrars or cancer registrars in the USA, and data collectors and multidisciplinary team coordinators in the UK—sometimes have difficulty because of the richness of the English language and the number of terms borrowed from Latin, Greek, and other languages. It takes either a good teacher or a good reference book to explain, for example, that the internal mammary lymph nodes and the parasternal lymph nodes are actually the same chain of lymph nodes, but are identified by different names in different medical specialities.

Cancer data collectors have earned the respect of their health-profession peers because they are performing a detailed, highly technical job, even though they are largely self-taught. Most cancer data collectors do not have medical degrees or extensive training in anatomy and physiology, yet they must be able to recognize a variety of oncology terms and know whether those terms are synonymous or different, so that they can record the stage of the cancer and the primary site and cell type with precision. Such precision is necessary for tracking cancer treatments for individual patients, analyzing epidemiologic studies and planning national cancer control efforts. In fact, a certification examination is offerred by the National Cancer Registrars Association in the USA to document a data collector's level of experience and skill in cancer registration. Cancer data collectors throughout the world may take the examination, which tests knowledge of coding and staging, anatomy and physiology, the cancer disease process, and the epidemiology of cancer. Most of the content is covered in this book, *Notes on Anatomy and Oncology*.

I initially became involved with this book when I was asked by the publisher to be an impartial anonymous reviewer of a book proposal developed by David O'Halloran. My name happened to be taken from a list on a cancer information website in the USA. What a coincidence that was, because I have been training registrars and writing reference materials for cancer data collectors in the USA for many years. I responded that a pocket reference that included information on anatomy, physiology, epidemiology, staging and treatment of cancer was a good idea and that there is definitely a need for this type of book in any English-speaking cancer registry. The proposal was accepted, the content was developed and edited, and ultimately I was invited to write this foreword.

David and his colleagues, Kathryn Guyers and Jill Henderson, based these *Notes* on the class materials they have used to train and educate data collectors for the registries and cancer networks throughout the UK. They understand what is pertinent to determining the primary site of the cancer, the cell type, the stage, and the appropriate treatment for various types of cancers, and they remained focused on conveying that information throughout the chapters of this book.

*Notes on Anatomy and Oncology* is both useful and important to cancer data collectors for several reasons. First, the content has been written for cancer data collectors—not nurses, medical students, general physicians, or oncology specialists, as so many cancer reference books are. For that reason alone, this book is unusual and highly desirable.

Secondly, the descriptions of the many locations where a cancer can arise are presented as regional anatomy, not functional or systemic anatomy. In other words, it is necessary for a cancer data collector to know what organs, perhaps in other body systems, are adjacent to the cancer site, as well as the lymphatic drainage of the cancer site, in order to properly determine the extent of the cancer spread. This regional anatomic presentation is another unique feature of this book. Many of the anatomic illustrations using this concept were created especially for this book.

Thirdly, a self-taught person learns best when the reasons behind the information or procedure are explained. *Notes on Anatomy and Oncology* includes sufficient organ physiology that the reader can understand why a particular cancer spreads in the way that it does, but without becoming a text on physiology. The book also includes enough epidemiology so that the reader can understand why a particular cancer is prevalent or has an unsatisfactory prognosis. In addition, because it is intended for both self-instruction and the classroom setting, the authors have included questions at the end of each section to evaluate the comprehension of the reader.

Fourthly, the cancer information presented is state-of-the-science. The primary staging reference is the sixth edition of the *AJCC Cancer Staging Manual*, which was published in 2002 by the American Joint Committee on Cancer. To my knowledge, this is the first registrar-oriented reference book (other than the staging manual itself) to incorporate the newest definitions of the tumor–node–metastasis (TNM) system of describing cancer stage. Furthermore, the section on the blood and lymphatic systems describes the most recent re-classification of these diseases, published by the World Health Organization in 2000. Even the facts cited in the various chapters are based on the most recent data analyses available.

Finally—and certainly not of least importance—the book speaks the language of physicians in terms that non-physicians can understand, providing a cross-pollination of terminology and cancer information of value to registries on both sides of the Atlantic. Both UK and US terminology is included when there is a difference. The better a cancer data collector understands what he or she reads in the health record, the more likely it is that the data collected will be accurate and useful.

For all of these reasons, I believe that *Notes on Anatomy and Oncology* provides a remarkable reference for cancer data collectors. With this tool, they and the health professionals creating the medical records are no longer separated by their common langauge.

Gaithersburg 2004 April G. Fritz

# Preface

Oncology, the study of cancer, is a field that is forever developing and one of the most rapidly changing of all medical specialties. It is also a specialty that is at the forefront of many lay people's thinking, be they politicians, cancer patients, or members of the general public concerned about cancer prevention, and very often finds itself at the top of governmental 'to do' lists. Many areas of the world endeavor to collect detailed and accurate information on the incidence and distribution of cancer cases, as well as information on treatment efficacy and mortality rates. However, the people who are relied upon to collect these data tend to have little or no background, either educational or clinical, in cancer as a disease. The changing roles and responsibilities of personnel working in the area of collection and collation of cancer data mean that in the future they will be required to have detailed knowledge of cancer as a disease.

*Notes on Anatomy and Oncology* has arisen from the authors' many years of experience of lecturing to people who deal with cancer, cancer data and cancer information in all its guises. Many of the books on the market cover oncology very well but tend to be very detailed. Readers without an already extensive knowledge of the subject can lose interest. While successfully delivering courses on anatomy and oncology to staff from cancer registries and cancer networks throughout the UK, we felt that the time was right to set down that learning experience in text. This book relates oncology to specific anatomy, something that we realize must be grasped by learners if they are to begin to understand why malignancies occur in certain places.

We have written this book specifically with those in mind who work in the collection, collation and use of cancer data and information. It will be of particular use to people working in this field who may have no previous clinical background, for example employees of cancer registries, clinical coders, multidisciplinary team (MDT) coordinators and medical secretaries. *Notes on Anatomy and Oncology* will also be of interest to those studying cancer as part of their education and training, for example student therapeutic radiographers, oncology nurses and medical students. If specialists in the field of cancer find the information in this book useful, then we are honored. However, it is not primarily aimed at such professionals, as there are many other, more specialized texts on the market which suit their needs.

We have attempted to allow the reader to simply and easily digest the information required for the study of cancer. Our aim is to explain the relationship between anatomy and oncology in a clear and concise way. The book has several unique features which makes it a useful learning tool for the reader as well as a useful reference text. It begins by introducing the reader to the basic concepts of cancer formation. It does this by providing an introduction to cell biology and highlights how a normal cell becomes abnormal, resulting in cancer. It develops this further by taking each body system and relating the anatomy and oncology specific to that area of the body. Each area of oncology covered incorporates the latest tumor–node–metastasis (TNM) classification* for that particular disease and, in particular, the book highlights the latest World Health Organization thinking on lymphomas and leukemias. Readers will find at the end of each chapter a series of self-assessment questions to test their learning on specific areas.

Leeds 2004

D. O'Halloran
K. Guyers
J. Henderson

---

* Unless specified otherwise, all TNM information herein is reproduced or adapted from the sixth edition of the *AJCC Cancer Staging Manual*, compiled by F L Greene et al. and published by Springer in New York and Heidelberg/Berlin. The equivalent UICC publication is *TNM Classification of Malignant Tumours*, 6th edn, edited by L H Sobin and Ch Wittekind and published by Wiley in Chichester and New York.

# Acknowledgments

We are well aware that no small group of people can be experts in all branches of oncology. We have attempted in this text to bring together our combined years of experience in both clinical and academic settings. We have been privileged to meet many people along the way, not least those clinical coders, MDT coordinators, clinical audit staff, medical secretaries, researchers (you know who you are!) and others from whom we have learned a great deal which has helped us to put this book together. We are greatly indebted to April Fritz, from the National Cancer Institute, Bethesda, Maryland, USA, whose knowledge of the subject is immense. Without April's help this book would not have been written, and for this we thank her. Also, an acknowledgment is due to the publishers, Elsevier, without whose backing, and probably greater strategic thinking, this book would not have evolved.

Any thanks would not be complete if we were not to mention our loved ones who have helped us all with ideas, practical support and generally kind words of encouragement.

We also, by means of this publication, want to pay special thanks to a person who, although not directly involved in its writing, was hugely influential in the personal and professional development of each of the authors. Chris Sharkey unfortunately passed away in September 1999, and she is sorely missed. Her mentoring throughout the years gave us the confidence to work at the highest levels. Hers was the original idea to teach anatomy and oncology to non-clinicians. Thirteen years on, the course is still running strongly throughout the UK! Chris, we thank you for all the support you gave us and we are glad to have been your colleagues and friends.

Leeds 2004

D. O'Halloran
K. Guyers
J. Henderson

# 1

# Introduction: what is cancer?

Cancer is not one but many diseases, which makes it difficult to define. However, there are some important similarities among all the different types of cancer, which together begin to build a picture of what cancer is:

- Cancer manifests itself as a neoplasm, or new growth.
- Cancer results from uncontrolled proliferation of body cells.
- This uncontrolled proliferation is caused by some form of mutation within the genes of the cell itself.
- This mutation is caused by genetic instability that is the result of exposure to carcinogens.
- Even if the stimulus that evoked the mutation and change is removed, the neoplasm will continue to grow.

In order to understand how cancer forms and develops, it is necessary to take a look at what makes up a normal body.

## THE CELL

The basic unit of life is the cell, a complex universe in miniature. A basic understanding of the relationship between the process of cancer and the anatomy of the body will be useful. Cells have many functions, and contain many specialized structures called *organelles* that carry out essential processes. Table 1.1 summarizes the major organelles of the cell and their functions.

**Table 1.1**  Summary of the most important cell constituents (not comprehensive)

| Name of organelle | Structure | Function | Oncological implications |
|---|---|---|---|
| Nucleus | Usually a round body; surrounded by nuclear membrane with pores for transport in and out; composed of nucleoplasm and chromatins | Control center of cell, responsible for replication | Source of genetic material; if wrong instructions, mutations can occur, possibly leading to tumor development |
| Plasma membrane/ cell membrane | Membrane made of lipid and protein; gives structure to cell | Allows movement of substances of certain sizes into and out of the cell; limits size and gives structure to cell; if membrane is ruptured, then cell is not viable | Cells lose their normal cell inhibition; leads to build-up of cells (proliferation); may lead to tumor growth |
| Protoplasm (in cell known as cytoplasm; in nucleus known as nucleoplasm) | Complex living material; semi-fluid, consists of water, chemicals, proteins, organic molecules, fats, etc. | | Change in expected ratio of nucleus size (N) to amount of cytoplasm (C) can indicate carcinogenic changes: normal mature cells have a low nucleocytoplasmic ratio (N:C); many tumor cells have a high N:C ratio |
| Nucleolus | Dark spherical mass within nucleus | Synthesizes proteins | Inappropriate proteins may or may not be produced |
| Centrosome | Small spherical structure close to nucleus; contains two dark granules called centrioles | Essential for early stages of cell division; forms structure to support division | Any mutations in the cell may disrupt normal cell division |
| Chromatin masses/ threads | Not normally seen unless division is to take place; they then thicken and become visible as individual threads known as chromosomes | As thickened threads, chromosomes composed of helical double chains of deoxyribonucleic acid (DNA) carry genes that are essential for heredity | Any interference in synthesis of DNA can cause the development of tumors; radiotherapy and chemotherapy can be effective as the cell is very sensitive at this phase |
| Vacuoles | Clear spaces within cytoplasm that can move and align with membrane to expel products | Transport waste substances or cell-produced secretions out of the cell | If the cell is undergoing carcinogenic changes, may export or import inappropriate substances |

Each cell is surrounded by a membrane that separates it from other cells and from the external environment (Fig. 1.1). This is known as the *plasma membrane (cell membrane)*. It is very thin, between 6 and 10 nanometers (or 6–10 millionths of a millimeter in thickness). Until the introduction of the electron microscope it could not be seen. This plasma membrane is a complex sandwich of phospholipid (lipid means fatty) layers and proteins with holes or pores that act as gateways and allow only certain substances in and out of the cell. These gateways are referred to as semi-permeable.

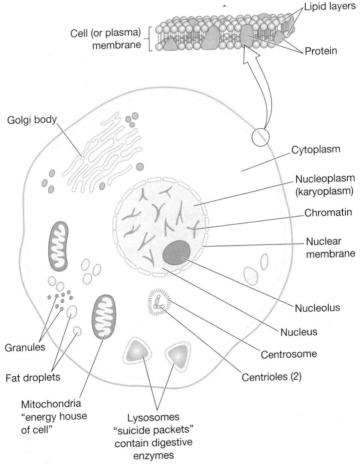

**Figure 1.1**   Major components of the cell.

Usually the plasma membrane is freely permeable to water, but its permeability to other substances seems to depend on several factors, including:

- *The size of the molecule*—large molecules cannot pass through; water and amino acids are small molecules, so they pass through the plasma membrane easily. Proteins are amino acids linked together, and many are very long, so they are too big to pass through.
- *Solubility in lipids*—substances that dissolve easily in lipids pass through the membrane more readily than other substances.
- *Charge of ions*—the charge of an ion trying to cross the plasma membrane can determine how easily that ion enters or leaves the cell. The protein part of the membrane is capable of being ionized. If an ion has a charge opposite to that of the membrane, it is attracted to the membrane and passes through more readily. If the ion has the same charge as the membrane, it is repelled and it cannot pass through.
- *Presence of carrier molecules*—plasma membranes contain special molecules called carriers that attract and transport substances across the membrane regardless of size, ability to dissolve in lipids, or charge of the membrane.

## Cytoplasm

Inside the plasma membrane surrounding the cell is a thick, semi-transparent, elastic fluid called cytoplasm. This is where many of the cell's organelles are found. Chemically, cytoplasm is 75–90% water plus solid components: proteins, carbohydrates, lipids and inorganic substances. This is where chemical reactions occur. The cytoplasm receives raw materials from outside the cell and converts them into useable energy. The cytoplasm is where new substances are created (synthesized), and it also packages chemicals for transport to other parts of the cell or to other cells.

## Nucleus

Central to the control and functioning of the cell is the nucleus, which is responsible for cell growth, metabolism and reproduction. The nucleus is usually a round or oval organelle bounded by a membrane called the *nuclear membrane*. It is the largest structure in the cell. Changes in the shape and size of the nucleus are known as *nuclear pleomorphism* and may indicate the cell is undergoing neoplastic change. Within the nucleus is a *nucleolus*, which is essential for cell division and contains the structures called chromosomes, of which there are 46 in a (diploid) human cell. Chromosomes are complex, but are basically composed of proteins and DNA (deoxyribonucleic acid) which carries genetic information representing a blueprint for protein synthesis. Genes are blocks of the chromosomal DNA chains, arranged in a specific sequence on the chromosomes. Genes determine the characteristics of the cell. Chromosomes also control cell structure and direct many of the cell's activities. Chromosomes contain all the genetic material essential for life; for example, in some very specialized cells (nerve cells), the absence of a centrosome (contains centrioles and is found in the nucleus—see section on mitosis) means the cell cannot divide, which is why nerve cells cannot be replaced if destroyed. Furthermore, since the cells cannot divide, they do not tend to develop into malignant neoplasms. In order to understand how cancer develops, it is important to consider how these genes affect the life cycle of the cell.

## THE CELL CYCLE (see Fig. 1.2)

Most of the organelles mentioned maintain the function of the cell on a day-to-day basis. However, during a human lifetime, millions and millions of cells are produced and millions are lost as cells are damaged, die, or are destroyed. New cells are produced to replace them, so the overall number remains in a stable state, keeping the cell population in equilibrium. It is estimated that, in 2 hours, 4 million red blood cells die and 4 million grow to replace the lost cells. To maintain the normal balance of cell numbers, cells have to go through a cell cycle where they duplicate all cell organelles and chromosomes, so that at the end of the cycle the result of division is two identical daughter cells.

Before a cell enters the cell cycle in preparation for division, it is said to sit in a phase called $G_0$. This is the 'resting phase' where cells will only be called upon to enter the cell cycle as a result of chemical stimulation. The impetus to enter the cycle is controlled by specialized genes and proteins, and after one cycle the cell may return to $G_0$. The true cycle consists mainly of two major periods: *interphase*, when a cell is not dividing, and the *mitotic* phase (mitosis), when a cell is dividing.

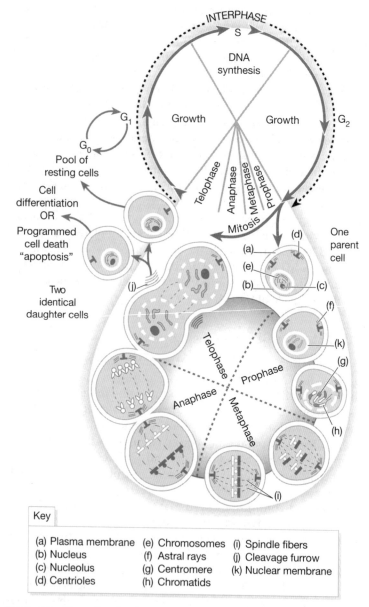

**Figure 1.2** The cell cycle, showing phases of mitosis.

Interphase is a relatively long process, during which the cell replicates DNA and additional organelles and other components are synthesized in preparation for mitosis. It is a frantic time, full of activity, with the cell doing most of its growing in this state. Interphase comprises three phases: $G_1$, S, and $G_2$. The $G_1$ phase is the initial growth phase where the cell enters the cycle from $G_0$. During $G_1$, there is a high level of metabolic activity. The cell duplicates most of its organelles and cytoplasmic components, but not DNA. If the cell cycle were 24 hours long, $G_1$ would last 8–10 hours. The duration of this phase is quite variable—in cancer cells, it might be very short. Once $G_1$ is complete the cell proceeds to the next phase, S-phase. The S (synthesis) phase would last about 8 hours, during which DNA replication occurs. When DNA replicates, some of its structure partly uncoils and other parts remain coiled; the uncoiled portion stains darker than coiled portions. This uneven distribution of stain causes DNA to appear as a granular mass called chromatin. As DNA uncoils, it forms a new strand alongside the original strand so that there are two DNA molecules. The cell also produces most of its RNA (ribonucleic acid). As interphase progresses, a pair of centrioles appears. Once a cell enters S phase, it is committed to go through cell division. During this process the cell acquires specialized biochemical properties such as cell surface proteins, chemical synthesis, or hormone responses. The $G_2$ phase or secondary growth phase would last 4–6 hours, during which cell growth continues.

Once a cell has achieved a duplicate content of organelles and DNA, it is ready to enter the mitotic phase—cell division. Ultimately the cell will divide to become two cells. One of these will return to the $G_0$ phase to be called on again if necessary. The other cell will *differentiate* into the type of cell its chromosomes designed it to be.

## NORMAL CELL DIVISION

In normal cells, cell division can be of two kinds: mitosis and meiosis.

### Mitosis

Mitosis is a process whereby a single parent cell duplicates itself. This process ensures that the two daughter cells are produced with the same number and identical chromosomes as the parent cell.

After the process, the two daughter cells possess the same heredi-tary material and genetic potential as the parent cell. This kind of cell division results in an increase in cell number, so that dead and injured cells can be replaced and new cells added for body growth.

Mitosis is divided into four stages (see Fig. 1.2). This is an arbi-trary classification as mitosis is a continuous process, one stage merging with another:

- *Prophase—the first phase of mitosis.* The centrioles move apart and project a series of radiating fibers. The centrioles move to opposite poles of the cell and become connected by another sys-tem of fibers called spindle fibers. Together they are called the mitotic apparatus. Simultaneously the chromatin shortens into chromosomes. The nucleoli become less distinct and the nuclear membrane disappears. The chromosome is composed of a pair of structures called chromatids; each chromatid is attached to its pair by a small body called the centromere. During prophase the chro-matid pairs (23 pairs) move towards the equator of the cell.
- *Metaphase—lining up.* The chromatid pairs line up on the equator of the cell. The centromere of each chromatid pair attaches itself to a spindle fiber.
- *Anaphase—dividing.* The centromeres divide and the identical sets of chromatids, now called chromosomes, have finished moving to opposite poles of the cell. During this movement, the centromeres attached to the spindle fibers seem to drag the trailing parts of the chromosomes toward opposite poles.
- *Telophase—the final phase.* New nuclear membranes begin to form around the sets of chromosomes; the chromosomes start to assume their chromatin form. Nucleoli reappear, spindle fibers disappear. The centrioles also replicate, so each cell has two cen-triole pairs. The formation of two identical nuclei to those of inter-phase terminates the telophase. *Cytokinesis* is the division of the cytoplasm. Cytokinesis begins in late anaphase with the forma-tion of a cleavage furrow that extends around the cell's equator. The furrow progresses inwards, resembling a constricting ring, eventually cutting through the cell to form two separate portions of cytoplasm, and finishes at the same time as telophase.

## Meiosis

Meiosis is cell division which results in germ cells (sperm and ova) being produced. This process allows the reproduction of an

**Table 1.2**    The relationship between germ layers and developing tissues

| Germ layer of embryo | Specific tissues derived from germ layer |
|---|---|
| Ectoderm (outer layer) | Forms the epithelium—skin, hair, nails, and lining of the glands that open onto the skin surface, the majority of the nervous system, and the epithelium of nose, sinuses, roof of the mouth, gums, cheeks, and the lower part of the anal canal |
| Mesoderm (middle layer) | Forms all connective and skeletal tissues, muscles, blood, blood vessels and lymphatic vessels, the urinary (except bladder and urethra) and reproductive systems |
| Endoderm (inner layer) | Forms the epithelial linings of the pharynx, thyroid and alimentary canal, glands that open into the alimentary canal, respiratory tract, the majority of the urinary bladder and urethra |

entirely new organism. The normal number of chromosomes is halved, so that when an ovum is fertilized by a sperm, the resulting embryo will have the normal complement of chromosomes and will possess the characteristics of both the mother and the father. The resulting embryo develops from a single fertilized cell that will go on to develop three germ layers, known as *ectoderm, mesoderm,* and *endoderm.* From these three germ layers develop all tissues and organs found in the mature adult (see Table 1.2).

## TISSUES

A tissue is a group of similar cells that, with their intercellular substance, function together to perform a specific activity, such as protection and support, producing chemicals (enzymes and hormones), or moving food through organs. Tissues can be grouped into several major categories: for example, epithelial, connective, muscular and nervous tissue.

There are four basic tissues of the body:

- general supporting tissues, collectively called the *mesenchyme*: connective tissue, with fibroblasts which form collagen fibers and associated proteins for bone, cartilage, muscle, blood vessels, and lymphatic vessels
- organ-specific cells: epithelium and specific cells for specific organs such as skin, intestine, liver
- defense cells: reticuloendothelial cells are a wide group of cells derived mainly from precursor red and white cells in the bone marrow; some cells are distributed about the body as free

cells and others as fixed organs such as lymph nodes and spleen

- nervous system: central nervous system (brain and spinal cord) and peripheral nervous system.

## Epithelial tissue

Epithelial tissue covers body surfaces, lines body cavities, and forms glands (see Fig. 1.3 and Table 1.3). Epithelium forms the outer covering of the body and some internal organs. It lines the body cavities and the interiors of the respiratory tract, gastro-intestinal tract, blood vessels and ducts. The epithelium forms the body's surface (skin), the surfaces of body cavities and their vis-cera, glands, and all tubular organs, including ducts and vessels. Epithelial tissue is arranged in single (simple) or several (strati-fied) layers; the cells are held together by specialized fibers and substances (for example, a basement membrane). Epithelial tissue can be sensitive to stimuli, such as taste and smell, but is avascu-lar (has no blood supply) and receives nutrition by diffusion.

Normal features of epithelial tissue include the following:

- Cells are closely packed.
- There is little or no intercellular material (matrix).
- Cells are in continuous sheets, single or multilayered.
- Nerves may extend through the sheets, but blood vessels do not.
- Vessels that supply nutrition and remove waste (blood and lymphatics) lie in underlying connective tissue.

Epithelium overlies and closely adheres to connective tissue. The junction between the connective and epithelial tissues is a thin extracellular layer called the *basement membrane*, from which epithelial layers develop. In malignant epithelial neoplasms, pen-etration of the tumor through the basement membrane gives the tumor the potential to spread to other parts of the body.

## Connective tissue

Connective tissue derives from mesenchyme cells which have broken away from the embryonic mesoderm. These *mesenchymal* cells distribute themselves throughout the three germ layers of the embryo (see Table 1.2), becoming the most abundant tissue in the body. Some mesenchymal cells remain in an undifferentiated

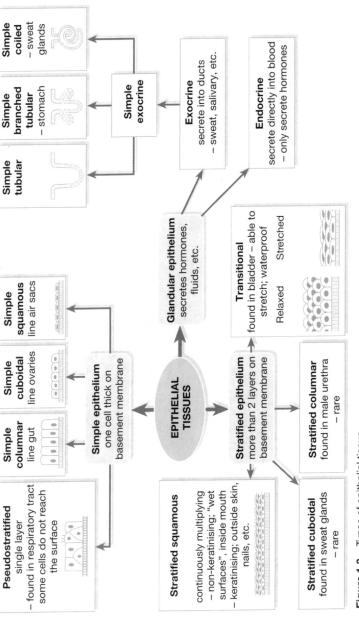

**Figure 1.3** Types of epithelial tissue.

**Table 1.3** Classification of normal epithelial tissue

| Epithelial tissue | Cell shape | Appearance | Arrangement and function |
|---|---|---|---|
| Simple | Squamous | Flat, scale-like, often described as pavement-like | Single layers; delicate; found in areas of absorption and filtration; occurs where there is little wear and tear |
| | Cuboidal | Cube-like | |
| | Columnar | Rectangles set on end | |
| Stratified | Squamous | As above | Made of at least two layers, that can withstand wear and tear |
| | Cuboidal | | |
| | Columnar | | |
| | Transitional | A combination of shapes: a bottom layer of cuboidal or columnar, a middle layer of cuboidal, and a superficial layer of cuboidal or squamous epithelium that allows expansion and can be waterproof, e.g. bladder | |
| Pseudostratified | Squamous | Appears as many-layered cells | Single layer but appears multilayered; not all cells are in contact with outer surface |
| | Cuboidal | | |
| | Columnar | | |
| Glandular (secretory) | Squamous | Classified structurally | Single or groups of epithelial cells which produce secretions, e.g. hormones, saliva, enzymes |
| | Cuboidal | Simple ducts or compound ducts that are branched, e.g. gastric and uterine | |
| | Columnar | Coiled tubular, e.g. sweat glands | |

state in the adult but the majority differentiate into cells that share a number of characteristics. As the name suggests, connective tissue serves as a connecting system, binding all other tissues together (see Fig. 1.4). Connective tissue can be categorized as bone tissue, which includes cartilage, and soft tissue, which can be embryonic, muscular, nervous, fat or fibrous (see Table 1.4). Its functions are to bind, protect, and support organs. Connective tissue has a rich blood supply; in other words it is highly vascular, except for cartilage, which is avascular.

Features of normal connective tissue:

- Cells are widely scattered within large quantities of an intercellular substance referred to as the *matrix;* the cells of the tissue secrete this.
- The matrix of the tissue determines the qualities of the tissue, e.g. fluid, semi-fluid, or mucoid.
- Cartilage is a connective tissue, but its matrix is firm and pliable. The matrix of bone is hard and not pliable.
- The cells also store fat, ingest bacteria and cell debris, form anticoagulants, and create antibodies to protect the tissue from disease.

## NEOPLASMS

Sometimes cells undergo duplication outwith the normal control mechanisms of the body. This can result in an excess of new tissue, called a *neoplasm* or tumor. The study of tumors is called *oncology.* Normal cell replication is under careful control in the body. To ensure that a cell is initiated and stimulated through the cycle, there are a number of specialized cellular proteins that support the phases of the cell cycle:

- *Proto-oncogenes* encourage and promote growth and division of cells as a response to signals from other cells. This involves relaying information from the cell membrane to the nucleus via the cytoplasm. If these proto-oncogenes are damaged, perhaps by a carcinogen or virus, they can mutate and become *oncogenes,* which promote overproduction of growth factors and uncontrolled cell growth. About a hundred oncogenes have been recognized to date (for example, the *ras, myc, neu, src,* and *sis* oncogenes).
- *Tumor suppressor genes* act as guardians for the cell, monitoring any mutations. At certain points within the cell cycle, the cell will

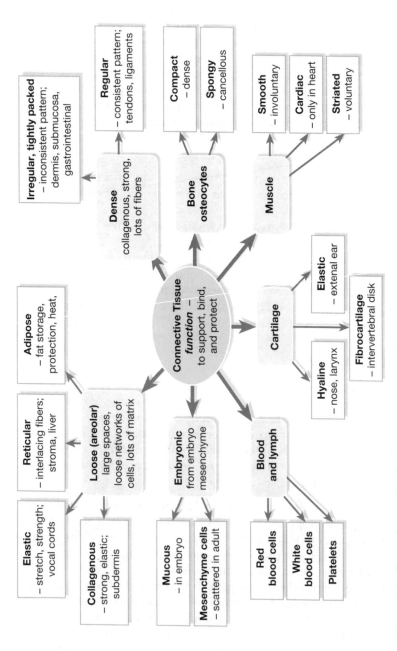

**Figure 1.4** Types of connective tissue.

**Table 1.4** Classification of normal connective tissue

| Name | Description | Examples |
|---|---|---|
| Loose or areolar | Jelly-like substance contains cells and loose network of fibers | Subcutaneous connective tissue |
| Adipose | Similar to areolar but cells store fat | Deposits around the kidneys |
| Dense fibrous | Fibers predominate | |
| | —Regularly arranged | Tendons, ligaments, elastic ligaments |
| | —Irregularly arranged | Dermis |
| Reticular | A network of fine branching reticular fibers supporting cells of organs | Spleen, liver |
| Cartilage | A firm plastic matrix containing fibers | |
| | —Hyaline is translucent, with fine collagen fibers | Cartilage of trachea |
| | —Fibrocartilage is dense, with collagenous fibers embedded in matrix | Intervertebral disks |
| | —Elastic cartilage has elastic fibers embedded in matrix | Cartilage of pinna, epiglottis |
| Bone | Solid, rigid matrix containing collagenous fibers | |
| | —Compact bone formed of Haversian systems (osteons) | Shaft of long bones |
| | —Spongy or cancellous bone; network or trabeculae of bone tissue between bone-marrow-filled cavities | Epiphyses of long bones |
| Dentine | Matrix similar to bone | Teeth |
| Hemato-poietic | Myeloid Lymphatic | Red marrow of ribs Spleen, lymph nodes |

effectively check itself to see that everything is in order before it proceeds to the next phase of the cycle. Tumor suppressor genes are responsible for this checking process, and they stimulate the cell to kill itself if there is a possibility that cell division may result in some form of mutation. This programmed cell death is called *apoptosis* (see Fig. 1.2). If tumor suppressor genes are mutated, the cell effectively becomes immortal, allowing continuous division of a mutated cell to occur. Tumor suppressor genes that are lost or inactivated can be a common prelude to cancer or tumor development. For example, in over 50% of all tumors, the tumor suppressor gene *p53* is damaged.

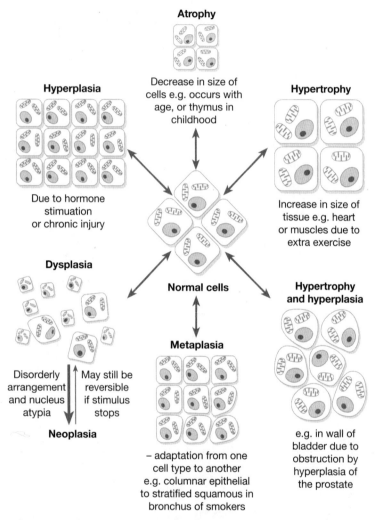

**Figure 1.5** Cellular changes from normal to abnormal states.

There are a number of disorders which constitute abnormal cell growth:

- *Hyperplasia* is an increase in the number of cells. There may also be an increase in the size of the cells, often a response to cell damage or destruction or increased hormone stimulation.
- *Dysplasia* is disordered growth and may indicate a change in cell shape, growth, or differentiation (see Fig. 1.5). Low-grade

damage can result in tissue structure abnormalities and cell changes and can be a result of too many stimuli, such as infection, trauma, cytotoxic drugs, or radiation.

- *Neoplasia*, or new growth, results from a disorder of cell growth similar to that in hyperplasia (increase in cell number) but differs in that proliferation is uncontrolled.

## CANCER FORMATION (CARCINOGENESIS)

At times the body will overproduce cells (hyperplasia, see Fig. 1.5) because of normal growth processes: for example, enlargement of the uterus during pregnancy. However, if the stimulus is removed the overproduction stops and the cells return to normal. In cancer, however, the cells of the neoplasm continue to divide and grow. Cancer development or *carcinogenesis* is thought to be a 'multiple-hit process' whereby the cell accumulates damage. The more damaged the cell is, the more likely that proto-oncogenes will mutate into oncogenes that promote cell growth and division. At the same time, tumor suppressor genes can be damaged and become inactivated or lost, which allows mutated cells to continue to divide.

### Benign neoplasms

In benign tumors, there may be a few small mutations, but the cells will be cytologically identical to their tissue of origin (well differentiated) although they appear histologically as an overproduction of cells (hyperplasia). Benign tumors have a capsule that makes them relatively easy to remove. Benign tumors are not usually fatal. The exception is in the pituitary gland, where about 99% of tumors are benign but the site of the tumor (located in the sella turcica, a small depression in the bony plate in the base of the skull) makes it potentially life-threatening. As a pituitary tumor enlarges, the patient displays intracranial pressure symptoms that have fatal implications if not treated.

### Malignant neoplasms

Malignant neoplasms, on the other hand, usually have a central body with infiltrating projections that extend out to invade adjacent tissues. Malignant neoplasms are not held within a capsule, but will infiltrate locally and starve the normal adjacent tissue of its blood supply. Malignant neoplasms will eventually break

**Table 1.5**   Differences between benign and malignant neoplasms

| Benign | Malignant |
| --- | --- |
| Encapsulated | Not encapsulated |
| Grow by expansion and never invade. Produce pressure effects or systemic effects and may secrete hormones | Grow by expansion and invasion (direct spread) |
| Usually slow-growing | Growth rate can vary |
| Under some normal control of body | Under no control |
| Remain localized | Spread from primary site (metastasize) |
| Cells resemble original tissue—well differentiated | Cells have variety of presentations from well differentiated to very poorly differentiated (anaplastic) |
| Not usually fatal, unless pressing on a vital organ | Always fatal unless treated |

away and spread throughout the body, a process called *metastasis*. Metastatic cells are found in a distant organ and have not developed from the tissue of that organ. For example, if a breast cancer cell is found in the liver, cytologically it will resemble breast tissue. A summary of the differences between benign and malignant tumors is given in Table 1.5.

## Tumor growth

In normal tissue following a mitotic division (see Fig. 1.2), two identical daughter cells are produced. One daughter cell will stay available for cell division ($G_0$), and one cell will go on to develop into a mature cell with specialized structures and functions. This process where a cell changes and becomes specialized and mature is called *differentiation* and is a normal process that the majority of cells of the body will go through. There are some tissues that maintain the ability to divide throughout life—usually in an area under constant wear and tear that requires a constant supply of newly produced cells, such as the lining of the alimentary tract. As cells become more specialized they lose their ability to reproduce. Nerve cells are highly specialized and cannot reproduce; tumors of true nerve cells are extremely rare (although tumors known as gliomas do arise from cells called glial cells that support the nerve cells; see Chapter 4). Tumor cells, however, tend to divide more frequently than normal cells. Even within a single tumor, the rate of growth, the balance between tumor cell growth and tumor cell death, can vary enormously. This variable mitotic rate can result in different parts of the tumor demonstrating varied differentiation.

Differentiation suggests that the tumor cell looks like its parent cell. The less differentiated (poorly differentiated or *undifferentiated*) a cell is, the more mutated it is and the less like the parent tissue it looks and acts. Assessing the degree of differentiation is called *grading* and is defined as *'estimating the degree of malignancy'*. Also, a neoplasm's growth depends on its blood supply. A tumor that outgrows its blood supply can develop areas of *necrosis* (death) where cells have been starved of oxygen.

## MALIGNANT TUMORS

There are three major characteristics of malignant tumors:

- Their growth is not under normal parent tissue control.
- Their cells always show a degree of *anaplasia*—they are poorly differentiated, showing bizarre changes in the shape and size of the nucleus (*pleomorphism*) and a lack of resemblance to the cells of the parent tissue.
- They can *metastasize*. Malignant tumor cells can move away from the original site (primary) and travel to another site (secondary) in the body and grow there.

This ability to metastasize is the main difference between benign and malignant tumors and is the primary characteristic that makes the treatment of such tumors so problematic. In the majority of cases, metastasis—rather than the primary tumor—will be the cause of death. This process of metastasis begins with invasion of surrounding tissue (see Table 1.6). Normal cells arrange themselves in tissues in neat, orderly ways with 'their own personal space'. Growth of normal cells occurs until they touch another cell. At this point they stop: this is called *contact inhibition* and is a property that tumor cells ignore. The lack of contact inhibition enables malignant cells to invade in and around other tissues and starve the normal tissue of essential nutrients and oxygen, causing normal-cell death. Normal cells also demonstrate *cellular adhesion*: that is, cells of the same type clump together to form an organ or tissue. Malignant tumor cells lack cell adhesion, allowing them to break off from the primary tumor and invade other areas of the body. They may invade into cavities (abdominal

**Table 1.6** The spread of malignant neoplasms

| Type of spread | Description of spread |
|---|---|
| Direct or local | Variable growth patterns can result in the affecting of organ function. Ulceration, if on an epithelial surface, can produce perforation or a fistula (an abnormal passage formed between two related structures, such as the rectum and vagina). A tumor can cause obstruction or invade nerves, giving pain and symptoms far from the primary (for example, a Pancoast tumor of the upper lobe of the lung can cause arm pain by pressure on the brachial plexus (a concentrated group of spinal nerves that supply the arm) |
| By blood (hematogenous) | Tumor cells erode through blood vessels, travel throughout the bloodstream to distant sites, and form secondary tumors in organs with an abundant blood supply. Common tumors that spread via blood include lung, breast, thyroid, kidney, and prostate |
| By lymph (lymphatic) | Tumor cells erode through lymph channels, are carried along with the lymph, lodge in lymph nodes, and grow in the node as secondary tumors |
| Implantation (transcoelomic) | Tumor cells break off from the primary and spread throughout a body cavity via the fluid in the cavity, such as in the pleural, pericardial or peritoneal cavities, and implant on any surface in the cavity |
| Seeding | Tumor cells may be left in an incision after surgical intervention and may allow a recurrence of the primary tumor |

or thoracic) or erode through blood and lymph vessels and be carried away to distant parts of the body (see Table 1.6). Once lodged in other parts of the body (typically brain, lung, liver, or bone), the tumor cells are able to establish a new blood supply (*angiogenesis*) and thereby continue to grow. Eventually, unless an appropriate intervention is administered, the tumor will compromise the function of the organ it is in and cause organ failure, which may lead to death.

The time a cell takes to go through the cell cycle and produce two identical cells is called the *doubling time*. For an individual tumor, the doubling time can vary enormously. A neoplasm's growth is dependent on its blood supply, which initially involves starving the adjacent tissue as the tumor grows. Malignant tumors can secrete factors that cause angiogenesis. The rate of cell death divided by the number of cells with a blood supply is known as the *mitotic index*. Often by the time the neoplasm can be visualized by radiography (a mass approximately 0.5 cm in size), the monoclonal cell (meaning that all cells developed from one cell and are identical) will have gone through around 26 doublings, and this is often the

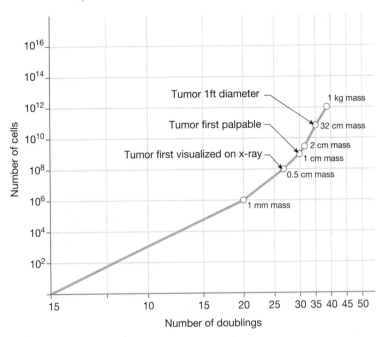

**Figure 1.6**   Tumor growth.

period of most rapid growth. The tumor may only require five to ten more doublings to grow from clinically palpable to systemic disease (see Fig. 1.6). In some cases, the neoplasm may become systemic before being clinically palpable, and the patient will present with metastatic disease from a *primary of unknown origin*.

Screening is a method whereby a malignancy can be detected before the disease becomes clinically apparent and produces symptoms. In the UK, there are two national screening programs, for breast cancer and cervical cancer, both of which have demonstrated the ability to detect cancers while they are still small and potentially more easily treated.

## CLASSIFICATION OF MALIGNANT TUMORS

Malignant tumors can be classified in a number of ways:

- histopathological
- locational
- biological
- descriptive.

**Table 1.7** Tumor terminology related to tissue of origin

| Tissue | Benign | Malignant |
|---|---|---|
| **Epithelium** | Papilloma | Carcinoma: |
| | | —basal cell carcinoma |
| | | —squamous cell carcinoma |
| | | —transitional cell carcinoma |
| Secretory or glandular epithelium | Adenoma | Adenocarcinoma |
| **Connective** | | Sarcoma |
| Bone | Osteoma | Osteosarcoma |
| Cartilage | Chondroma | Chondrosarcoma |
| Fat | Lipoma | Liposarcoma |
| Fibrous | Fibroma | Fibrosarcoma |
| Muscle, voluntary | Rhabdomyoma | Rhabdomyosarcoma |
| Muscle, involuntary | Leiomyoma | Leiomyosarcoma |
| **Fetal** | | ... blastoma |

## Histopathological

Tumors can be classified according to their tissue of origin (see Table 1.7):

- Tumors that develop from epithelial cells (found in skin and linings of the organs, digestive tract, and airways) are termed *carcinomas*. This is the most common cancer type, accounting for about 80–90% of all cancers.
- Tumors arising from connective tissues, such as muscle, bone, cartilage, and fat are termed *sarcomas*.
- Childhood tumors often occur if embryonic/fetal tissue is left behind. These tumors are named after the blastocytes from which cells and tissues are derived in the embryo: for example, nephroblastoma, neuroblastoma.
- Sometimes the tissue of origin cannot be determined as the cells are so undifferentiated. These tumors can then be classified as a primary of unknown origin.

## Locational

The actual site of any tumor is important in terms of symptoms, possible spread, treatment options, and even prognosis. Treatment options will be very different for a malignant melanoma of the retina than for a malignant melanoma on the forearm.

## Biological

Such a classification includes descriptions of the behavior of the tumor, such as:

- degree of differentiation (high, moderate, poor, anaplastic)
- whether lymphocytic reaction is present or absent, which gives an indication of whether the body is defending itself against the tumor
- hormone receptor status—some tumors, such as certain tumors of the breast, need hormones to survive; altering the body's hormonal environment may therefore be a useful treatment strategy
- degree of infiltration, especially involving blood vessels, which may provide an estimate of the likelihood of secondaries.

## Descriptive

Tumors can also be described by the way they look:

- *fungating,* where the tumor invades the epithelial surface, perhaps causing infection that may make the tumor resistant to treatments such as radiotherapy and chemotherapy
- *nodular,* where the tumor is hard and fibrous, which may indicate that the body is developing scar tissue in a response to disease; this may indicate a better prognosis for the patient
- *fixed* or *mobile*—if fixed (attached to other structures), this may indicate possible spread away from the primary site and a worse prognosis.

## Grade and stage

The classifications described above create an assessment of the tumor, which will affect the management options and prognosis of the patient. Tumors can also be categorized according to their *grade* and *stage.* All tumors derive from a single rogue cell. All subsequent cells should be identical or monoclonal; however, as the tumor cells continue to go through further cell cycles they continue mutating so that a range of differentiation may be present within a tumor. The proportion of undifferentiated cells defines the grade of the tumor and provides an estimate of the degree of malignancy.

**Table 1.8**  Relationship between tumor grade and prognosis

| Grade | Description | Prognosis |
|-------|-------------|-----------|
| 1 | <25% undifferentiated cells | Best |
| 2 | >25%, <50% undifferentiated | |
| 3 | >50%, <75% undifferentiated | |
| 4 | >75% undifferentiated | Worst |

### Grade

Generally grade is described on a scale of 1 to 4, as in Table 1.8. Sometimes a tumor can be so markedly undifferentiated that it is difficult to assess its tissue of origin. These are referred to as anaplastic tumors and are generally highly malignant, offering the worst prognosis.

### Stage

Staging is a way in which the characteristics of cancer can be described. It allows clinicians to relate individual cases to the human body. It can be described, therefore, as an anatomical classification of the disease. It is a measure of the size and extent of the tumor at the time of diagnosis. The uses of staging can be summarized as follows:

- Staging allows decisions to be made about the management of the cancer patient, identifying appropriate treatment(s).
- It allows similar cases to be compared, thus becoming a factor in estimating the prognosis of a case.
- Staging can aid in the development and evaluation of clinical trials, thereby allowing more effective management strategies to be developed.

The TNM (tumor–node–metastasis) staging system developed jointly by the Union Internationale Contre Le Cancer (UICC) and the American Joint Committee on Cancer (AJCC) is widely recognized around the world as the principal staging system for most types of cancer. TNM forms the basis for cancer data collection within the United Kingdom as part of the National Cancer Dataset and cancer data collection in cancer treatment facilities in the United States under the standards of the Commission on Cancer of the American College of Surgeons. Historically, there were many ways of staging different tumors, mainly dependent

**Table 1.9**   Some staging systems other than TNM

| Name of staging classification system | Tumors |
| --- | --- |
| Ann Arbor | Lymphomas (Hodgkin and non-Hodgkin) |
| Masaoka | Thymoma |
| FIGO | Female gynecologic cancers: ovary, vagina, endometrial, cervix |
| Dukes | Colorectal cancers |
| Royal Marsden Hospital | Testicular tumors |
| Jackson | Penile carcinoma |
| Reese | Retinoblastoma |

on the site within the body, which may lead to some confusion. Table 1.9 lists some of the other staging systems that may still be used for certain primary cancers.

TNM staging describes the anatomic extent of the tumor—that is, how localized or how far spread the tumor is. It does this on the basis of assessment of three components:

- T—extent of primary tumor
- N—absence or presence and extent of regional lymph node involvement by the tumor
- M—absence or presence of tumor at a distance from the primary site.

By assigning numbers to these components (typically 0–4), an indication of the extent or severity of the disease can be made.

The T component represents the primary tumor and its extent at the site of origin and can be classified according to the following general criteria:

- TX—minimum requirements to assess the primary tumor cannot be met
- T0—no evidence of primary tumor
- Tis—carcinoma in situ
- T1–T4—progressive increase in tumor size and/or involvement of other structures.

The definition of the T classification is relevant only for that particular tumor site and will vary from site to site. However, there are only two main ways in which tumor extension can be described: depth of invasion (e.g. bladder) and size of tumor (e.g. kidney).

The N component describes regional lymph node involvement and can be categorized according to the following:

- NX—minimum requirements to assess the regional lymph nodes cannot be met
- N0—no evidence of regional lymph node involvement
- N1–N3—increasing involvement of regional lymph nodes in size, number, location, or other factors.

It is important to note that the N category only applies to regional lymph nodes which are specifically listed in the sixth edition of the TNM staging manual. Involvement of other distant nodes is classified in the M category.

The M category describes the spread of the tumor via the blood to distant sites of the body:

- MX—minimum requirements for assessing the presence of distant metastases cannot be met
- M0—no evidence of distant metastases
- M1—presence of distant metastases.

Additional notations may be added to highlight the site of the metastases, such as PUL (pulmonary), HEP (liver), and BRA (brain).

Once the T, N and M categories have been noted, they are grouped to give a stage. Excluding the X category, there are 48 different permutations of these components: T (0–4, is), N (0–3) and M (0–1). These permutations are assigned to broader categories called *stage groups* to give an indication of likely prognosis and treatment strategy. For example, stage I indicates localized disease, and stage IV is advanced disease. Table 1.10 shows, for example, some aspects of how sarcomas (connective tissue tumors) are staged according to the TNM categories.

The classification of cancer, along with the stage and grade, forms the basis of an overall plan of treatment for a specific case. Such a treatment may use a combination of methods. The three main treatment strategies for cancer are surgery, radiotherapy, and chemotherapy. Other therapies, such as immunotherapy and hormone therapy also play an important role in the treatment of cancer.

## TREATMENT

To be effective against cancer, a treatment plan must take into consideration the stage of the disease. For example, early stage

**Table 1.10**  Example (for sarcomas) of cancer stage groups using the TNM classification[a]

| Stage | Primary tumor (T) | Regional node involvement (N) | Distant metastasis (M) |
|---|---|---|---|
| I | T1a, T1b, T2a, or T2b[b] | N0 | M0 |
| II | T1a, T1b, or T2a | N0 | M0 |
| III | T2b[b] | N0 | M0 |
| IV | Any T | N1 | M0 |
| | Any T | N0 | M1 |

[a] Note that grade (degree of differentiation) is also an important factor in assigning stage for sarcomas, as it reflects malignancy and has major implications for a patient's management and prognosis. The full TNM staging of sarcomas takes account of the grade of the tumor—see Table 3.2.
[b] For a low grade tumor, T2b indicates stage I; whereas, for a high grade tumor, it indicates stage III—see Table 3.2.

disease may be treated with a local treatment such as surgery, whereas later stage disease that has metastasized requires a more systemic approach to treatment, such as chemotherapy.

## Surgery

Surgery plays an important role in both the treatment of cancer and in diagnosis and staging. It is a 'local' treatment designed to remove all or part of the tumor at the primary site. Diagnostic samples (biopsies) can be removed and sent for further analysis to allow a histopathological diagnosis to be made. At the time of surgery, the surgeon may also sample lymph nodes to see if there is any involvement, thereby providing information for the N classification. The extent of the primary within the organ or tissue (T) can similarly be established.

Surgery, as a treatment modality, can control the primary tumor. It is also essential to recognize that many cancers may recur at the site of origin, making wide excision essential in some cases. Recognition of the role of other therapies such as radiotherapy has, however, led to a more conservative approach to some surgical techniques. In the early- to mid-1900s, breast cancer was traditionally treated using a radical or total mastectomy. Clinical trials in the 1970s and 1980s demonstrated that this may not always be necessary and that local excision of the tumor followed by radiotherapy to the breast could offer as good a chance of cure while keeping the breast intact.

## Radiotherapy

Radiotherapy is the treatment of cancer using high-energy radiation. It too is mainly a localized treatment, which can be broadly divided into two groups: teletherapy and brachytherapy.

*Teletherapy* (derived from the Greek words *tele*, meaning at a distance, and *therapeia*, meaning treatment) is also referred to as external beam radiotherapy. The radiation is created electronically by a linear accelerator. It is directed from a source outside the patient, the aim being for the radiation to traverse the patient and deposit its energy in the tissue and tumor. In order to get to deep-seated tumor sites, a radiation dose is also deposited in healthy tissues and this may lead to side effects such as epilation (local hair loss), erythema (reddening of the skin like sunburn), and mucositis (inflammation of the mucous membrane, for example, in the mouth).

*Brachytherapy* (Greek *brachys*: short range) is a medical treatment that involves the placement of small radioactive sources within a natural body cavity, within the tissues, or close to the surface. Whereas once the linear accelerator is switched off the radiation source disappears, this is not so with brachytherapy. The physics behind brachytherapy means that the radiation is deposited in a short range of tissue allowing very high doses to be given to the tumor without necessarily irradiating too much healthy tissue. Brachytherapy can be administered in a variety of ways:

- intracavity—the radioactive sources are placed into a cavity within the body, for example the uterus
- intraluminal—the radioactive sources are placed into a lumen of the body, for example the esophagus
- interstitial—the radioactive sources are placed through tissue, for example through the breast.

## Chemotherapy

Chemotherapy refers to the use of drugs to combat the disease process. More accurately, it should be referred to as cytotoxic chemotherapy because the drugs used to combat cancer have a cytotoxic (cell killing) effect. Chemotherapy drugs work by halting or disrupting the normal cell cycle (see Fig. 1.2). Different categories of drugs work in different ways, but essentially they stop DNA from forming or they somehow interact directly with it. Either way, the cell fails to replicate and therefore dies. Like radiotherapy, the chemotherapy drugs are non-discriminatory: that is, they affect healthy as well as tumor cells, and therefore side effects can occur. Generally speaking, the more frequently a cell is dividing, the more sensitive the cell is to the chemotherapy drug, which is why noted side effects tend to occur in those areas of the body with fast-dividing tissue (mucous membrane, digestive tract).

Both radiotherapy and chemotherapy rely on normal body cells repairing quicker than cancer cells, allowing for the destruction of the tumors, with the side effects disappearing over time. This is sometimes referred to as the *therapeutic ratio*.

### Immunotherapy

Immunotherapy is the name given to treatments that initiate the body to fight against the cancer. Immunotherapy drugs are sometimes referred to as biological response modifiers because they promote the body's own response to fight an infection (in this case cancer). Immunotherapy can be local, as in the treatment of carcinoma of the bladder, where BCG (bacillus Calmette–Guérin) is administered directly into the bladder via a catheter, or systemic, where the drug is used to treat the whole body, such as interferon or interleukin 2, which have been shown to be effective against kidney cancer. Moreover, immunotherapy drugs can be given to boost the body's natural defense system (termed non-specific immunotherapy) or they can be used to target individual tumor cells and not normal cells; the agents used in the latter case are called *monoclonal antibodies*.

## The multidisciplinary approach to the treatment of cancer

Much has been done over the past decade to bring groups of professionals together to work for the benefit of the individual cancer patient. Such groups are called 'multidisciplinary' teams. They comprise diverse disciplines that provide comprehensive assessment and consultation for a particular cancer case. While primarily there to help team members resolve difficult cases, teams may also fulfill a variety of additional functions. For example, they can help promote coordination between different professionals, provide a 'checks and balances' mechanism to ensure that the interests and rights of all concerned parties (particularly the patient) are addressed, and perhaps identify service gaps and breakdowns in coordination or communication. They also enhance the professional skills and knowledge of individual team members by providing a forum for learning more about the strategies, resources, and approaches used by various disciplines to the treatment of cancer. Such an approach to the treatment of cancer cases is essential for providing appropriate management strategies and attaining the best possible chance of cure for the patient.

## SELF-ASSESSMENT QUESTIONS

Answer true or false to the following. Answers are on page 243.

1. The outer layer of the cell is called the plasma membrane.
2. A well differentiated tumor is one that is unlike its parent tissue.
3. A tumor developing from epithelial tissue is given the term sarcoma.
4. Germ cells are formed by a process called mitosis.
5. All cells that are capable of division are able to become malignant tumors.
6. The grade of a tumor refers to its size and extent.
7. A benign tumor grows by extension and invasion.
8. A benign tumor does not metastasize.
9. There are three layers in the embryo, and the outermost layer is called the endoderm.
10. Malignant tumors can spread directly, by blood, lymphatics, across cavities and by seeding.
11. A benign tumor of fibrous tissue is called a fibroma.
12. Embryonal tumors develop from blast cells and are called blastomas.
13. Simple epithelial tissue has more than two layers.
14. Transitional epithelium has many layers so that it can expand.
15. The traditional staging system for gynecological tumors is the Dukes system.
16. Surgery plays an important role in the systemic treatment of cancer.
17. Transitional epithelium is found mainly in the skin.
18. The T classification in the TNM staging system involves the size of the tumor.
19. A classification of M1 suggests late stage disease.
20. Grade 4 suggests a well differentiated tumor.

# The circulatory systems: blood and lymph

The term circulatory system describes the cardiovascular and the lymphatic systems working together. Both consist of moving fluids necessary to transport essential minerals, proteins, gases, and other substances throughout the body. The vessels of the cardiovascular system form a closed circuit network that continually transports blood around the body. Lymphatic vessels, on the other hand, begin as blind-ended vessels within tissue spaces. Lymph is ultimately conveyed back into the blood via a series of lymphatic vessels.

## THE CARDIOVASCULAR SYSTEM

The cardiovascular system comprises the heart and blood vessels: namely, arteries, veins and capillaries (Fig. 2.1). The function of the heart is to pump blood around the body, and the blood is conveyed by arteries that generally take oxygenated blood away from the heart. Major arteries, such as the aorta, are responsible for the first part of this transportation. As the blood reaches organs or tissues where the oxygen is required, the arteries become ever smaller until ultimately they form capillaries that have walls one cell layer thick to enable the exchange of gases between the blood and tissue. Oxygen is absorbed into the tissue in exchange for carbon dioxide. This new blood, now without oxygen, transports carbon dioxide and other waste materials back towards the heart via small veins (venules) that join together to

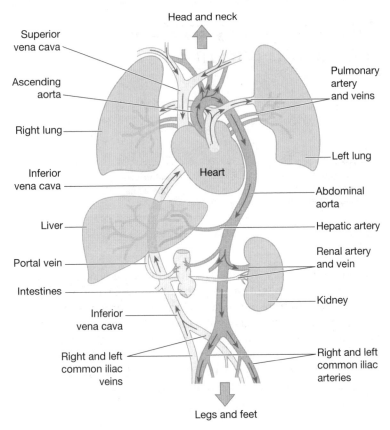

Head and neck

Superior
vena cava

Ascending
aorta

Right lung

Inferior
vena cava

Liver

Portal vein

Intestines

Inferior
vena cava

Right and left
common iliac
veins

Pulmonary
artery
and veins

Left lung

Heart

Abdominal
aorta

Hepatic artery

Renal artery
and vein

Kidney

Right and left
common iliac
arteries

Legs and feet

**Figure 2.1**   The flow of blood through major vessels.

form larger veins. The two largest veins in the body are the superior and inferior vena cava. The superior vena cava transports the blood from the head and neck area back toward the heart, and the inferior vena cava transports blood from the lower part of the body back to the heart.

## Blood

Blood is made up of blood cells (45%—red, white, and platelets) and plasma (55%). Plasma contains mainly water, proteins, gases, electrolytes, hormones, and other materials. The main function of the blood is to transport essential goods to tissues of the body and to transport waste material away from those tissues and out of the body.

Hematopoiesis (blood cell formation) takes place in the red bone marrow located in various parts of the body. In adults, red bone marrow can be found in the epiphyses of the humerus and femur, a few irregular or flat bones such as the vertebra, pelvic bones, and sternum, as well as in some lymphatic tissues, such as the lymph nodes, spleen, and thymus. The blood cells originate from *pluripotential stem cells*—that is, a single stem cell has the potential to differentiate into any of the types of blood cells. The differentiation pathway can be seen in Figure 2.2. It is important to recognize that the pluripotential stem cell, found at the beginning of the pathway, may proceed down either of two paths: the myeloid cell path or the lymphoid cell path. Each pathway will result in a variety of blood cells. The names of these cells and their functions can be found in Table 2.1. White cells, which can be further subdivided into granulocytes (those cells with granules in the cytoplasm) and agranulocytes (those without granules), play a major role in the body's immune response.

It is important to understand the pathway of blood cell differentiation in order to understand leukemias and lymphomas, the principal malignancies of the circulatory systems. Mutation of cells in the myeloid pathway may lead to myeloid diseases such as myeloid leukemia, whereas if the lymphoid pathway is affected then lymphoid disease such as lymphocytic leukemia or the lymphomas may result. In fact, the current thinking about the lymphoid differentiation pathway is that it is perhaps no longer suitable to separate out lymphocytic leukemias and lymphomas, as they are probably the same type of disease. The primary difference is that one manifests itself in the bone marrow and is termed leukemia, and the other manifests itself in the lymphatic system and is termed lymphoma. The World Health Organization (WHO) recognized this reorganization of traditional thinking in their classification of myeloid and lymphoid neoplasms (Table 2.2).

## THE LYMPHATIC SYSTEM

The lymphatic system is a specialized section of the circulatory system. Each organ in the body has an associated lymphatic drainage, the function of which is to return proteins, fats and other

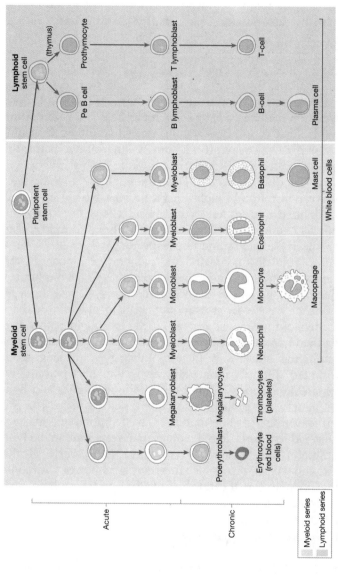

**Figure 2.2** The differentiation pathway for blood cells. Leukemias can develop from mutation of cells in either the lymphoid or the myeloid series. Mutation of cells early in the differentiation pathway tends to give rise to acute disease, whereas chronic disease tends to result if the affected cells are at an advanced stage of differentiation, as labeled here. Lymphomas arise from mutation of lymphoid cells.

**Table 2.1**   Blood cells and their function

| Differentiation pathway | Cell type | | Role/function |
|---|---|---|---|
| Lymphoid cells | Lymphocytes | Agranulocytes | T and B cells—major role in immune response; produce antibodies |
| Myeloid cells | Monocytes | Agranulocytes | Macrophages ingest microorganisms and detoxify cells |
| | Eosinophils | Granulocytes | Anti-inflammatory response; release chemicals to detoxify harmful products that accumulate as a result of infection |
| | Basophils | Granulocytes | Almost unknown; may release heparin to help prevent coagulation of the blood |
| | Neutrophils | Granulocytes | Migrate into tissue and ingest and digest microbes |
| | Erythrocytes (red blood cells) | | Carry oxygen around the body in the form of oxyhemoglobin, and return carbon dioxide to lungs to be excreted |
| | Thrombocytes (platelets) | | One of several clotting factors; assist in stopping bleeding |

substances from the tissues where they have been used back to the general circulation. The lymphatic system itself is made up mainly of lymphatic vessels that are similar in structure to veins, although their walls are thinner. These vessels originate as blind-ended vessels in tissue spaces and join together to form ever larger lymphatic vessels. All the lymph eventually drains into two major lymphatic vessels: the right lymphatic duct, which receives lymph from the upper right quadrant of the body, and the thoracic duct, which receives the rest of the body's lymphatic fluid. Lymph is finally returned to the blood via the right and left subclavian veins.

As lymph is transported throughout the body it travels through oval-shaped lymph nodes. Most lymph nodes are found in groups around the body (Fig. 2.3a). Lymph nodes are enclosed by a fibrous capsule. They receive lymph from a number of afferent

**Table 2.2** WHO classification of hematopoietic and lymphoid neoplasms

| Lineage | WHO term |
| --- | --- |
| **Myeloid neoplasms** | **Myeloproliferative diseases**<br>• Chronic myelogenous leukemia (CML), Philadelphia chromosome positive {t(9;22)(q34;q11)}, {*BCR/ABL*}<br>• Chronic neutrophilic leukemia<br>• Chronic eosinophilic leukemia/hypereosinophilic syndrome<br>• Chronic idiopathic myelofibrosis<br>• Polycythemia vera<br>• Essential thrombocythemia<br>• Myeloproliferative disease, unclassifiable<br><br>**Myelodysplastic/myeloproliferative diseases**<br>• Chronic myelomonocytic leukemia (CMML)<br>• Atypical CML<br>• Juvenile myelomonocytic leukemia<br><br>**Myelodysplastic syndromes**<br>• Refractory anemia<br>— With ringed sideroblasts<br>— Without ringed sideroblasts<br>• Refractory cytopenia (myelodysplastic syndrome) with multilineage dysplasia<br>• Refractory anemia (myelodysplastic syndrome) with excess blasts<br>• 5q– (5q deletion) syndrome<br>• Myelodysplastic syndrome, unclassifiable<br><br>**Acute myeloid leukemias (AMLs)**<br>*AMLs with recurrent cytogenetic translocations*<br>• AML with t(8;21)(q22;q22) {*AML1(CBF-alfa)/ETO*}<br>• Acute promyelocytic leukemia {*AML* with t(15;17)(q22;q11–12) and variants}, {*PML/RAR-alfa*}<br>• AML with abnormal bone marrow eosinophils {inv(16)(p13q22)} or {t(16;16)(p13;q11)}, {*CBFb/MYH11*}<br>• AML with 11q23 abnormalities {*MLL*}<br>• AML with multilineage dysplasia<br>— With prior myelodysplastic syndrome<br>— Without prior myelodysplastic syndrome<br>• AML and myelodysplastic syndromes, therapy-related<br>— Alkylating agent-related<br>— Epipodophyllotoxin-related (some may be lymphoid)<br>— Other types<br><br>**AML not otherwise categorized**<br>• AML minimally differentiated<br>• AML without maturation<br>• AML with maturation |

(*continued*)

**Table 2.2**   (continued)

| Lineage | WHO term |
| --- | --- |

- Acute myelomonocytic leukemia
- Acute monocytic leukemia
- Acute erythroid leukemia
- Acute megakaryocytic leukemia
- Acute basophilic leukemia
- Acute panmyelosis with myelofibrosis

**Acute biphenotypic leukemias**

**Lymphoid neoplasms**
*B cell neoplasms*

**Precursor B cell neoplasm**
- Precursor B lymphoblastic leukemia/lymphoma
- Precursor B cell acute lymphoblastic leukemia (ALL)

**Mature (peripheral) B cell neoplasms**
- B cell chronic lymphocytic leukemia (CLL)/small lymphocytic lymphoma
    —B cell prolymphocytic leukemia
    —Lymphoplasmacytic lymphoma
    —Splenic marginal zone B cell lymphoma
    —Hairy cell leukemia
- Plasma cell myeloma/plasmacytoma
    —Extranodal marginal zone B cell lymphoma of MALT type
    —Nodal marginal zone B cell lymphoma (with/without monocytoid B cells)
- Follicular lymphoma
    —Mantle-cell lymphoma
    —Diffuse large B cell lymphoma
    –Mediastinal large B cell lymphoma
    –Primary effusion lymphoma
- Burkitt lymphoma/Burkitt cell leukemia

**Hodgkin lymphoma (HL)**
- Nodular lymphocytic-predominant HL
- Classical HLs
    —Nodular sclerosis HL
    —Lymphocyte-rich classical HL
    —Mixed cellularity HL
    —Lymphocyte depletion HL

*T cell and natural killer cell neoplasms*

**Precursor T cell neoplasm**
- Precursor T lymphoblastic lymphoma/leukemia
- Precursor T cell ALL

**Mature (peripheral) T cell neoplasms**
- T cell prolymphocytic leukemia
- T cell granular lymphocytic leukemia
- Aggressive NK cell leukemia
- Adult T cell lymphoma/leukemia (HTLV-1 positive)
- Extranodal NK/T cell lymphoma, nasal type

(continued)

**Table 2.2** (continued)

| Lineage | WHO term |
| --- | --- |
| | • Enteropathy-type T cell lymphoma<br>• Hepatosplenic gamma–delta T cell lymphoma<br>• Subcutaneous panniculitis-like T cell lymphoma<br>• Mycosis fungoides/Sézary syndrome<br>• Anaplastic large cell lymphoma, T/null cell, primary cutaneous type<br>• Peripheral T cell lymphoma, not otherwise characterized<br>• Angioimmunoblastic T cell lymphoma<br>• Anaplastic large cell lymphoma, T/null cell, primary systemic type |
| **Mast cell diseases** | • Cutaneous mastocytosis<br>• Systemic mast cell disease<br>• Mast cell leukemia/sarcoma |
| **Macrophage/histiocytic neoplasm** | • Histiocytic sarcoma |
| **Dendritic cell neoplasms** | • Langerhans cell histiocytosis<br>• Langerhans cell sarcoma<br>• Interdigitating dendritic cell sarcoma/tumor<br>• Follicular dendritic cell sarcoma/tumor<br>• Dendritic cell sarcoma, not otherwise specified |

Only major disease categories are listed.
{ } indicates an alternative description of the neoplasm, involving the type of genetic mutation and/or the name of the gene implicated in the cause of the neoplasm.
HTLV, human T cell lymphotropic virus; MALT, mucosa-associated lymphoid tissue; NK, natural killer.
Adapted from: *International Classification of Diseases for Oncology*, 3rd edn, Table 13, pages 16–18. World Health Organization, Geneva, 2000.

vessels and allow lymph to leave the node via one or two efferent vessels (Fig. 2.3b). Valves within the lymphatic vessels allow the lymph to flow in one direction only. Trabeculae within the node form a fine meshwork of fibers which trap any harmful microorganisms contained within the lymph fluid. Throughout the cortex of the node are germinal centers that produce lymphocytes, which then act as a defense against any unwanted organisms caught within the framework.

In addition to the lymphatic vessels and lymph nodes, the body contains diffuse areas of lymphatic tissue called aggregated lymphatic nodules. These are primarily found where the body's internal environment is in contact with the external environment, for example in the digestive tract, where the tonsils and the aggregated lymphatic nodules in the stomach and intestines act as

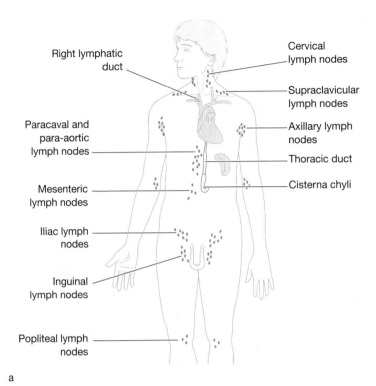

**Figure 2.3** (a) Distribution of lymph nodes; (b) a lymph node.

defenses against ingested pathogens. Lymphatic tissue can also be found in the lungs and the brain.

How organs drain via the lymphatic system is important in understanding the spread of cancer in general. The lymphatic spread of cancer can be traced by following the lymphatic flow, since lymph only flows in one direction. This is particularly important in the understanding of lymphomas, the general term to describe cancerous changes in lymphatic tissue.

## HEMATOPOIETIC MALIGNANCIES

The malignant hematopoietic diseases are a group of diseases characterized by the overproduction of blood cells, mainly white blood cells (see Table 2.3). As mentioned above, we distinguish myeloid neoplasms and lymphoid neoplasms. These can be further divided into two types: acute disease and chronic disease. Acute hematopoietic disease is typified by the presence of primitive blast cells in the bone marrow and peripheral blood. These cells are immature and at the beginning of the differentiation pathway shown in Figure 2.2. Chronic hematopoietic disease is associated with more mature cells that are further along the differentiation pathway but are still abnormal. The overproduction of these abnormal blood cells, again usually white cells, crowds out other blood cells, usually red blood cells and platelets. This leads to the common presenting symptoms such as anemia and a tendency to bleed or bruise easily. In hematopoietic disease, since only one type of white blood cell is being overproduced, other white blood cells, such as neutrophils, may be underproduced. Because of this, and also because the abnormal white blood cells do not function properly, the patient is susceptible to infection, which is one of the main causes of death, along with total bone marrow failure.

**Table 2.3** Normal and leukemic blood values

|  | Normal blood count | Leukemic blood count (approximate) |
| --- | --- | --- |
| Hemoglobin (Hg) | 10–14 g/dl | 7–9 g/dl |
| Total white cell blood count | $4$–$10 \times 10^9$/l | $10$–$200 \times 10^9$/l |
| Platelets | $250 \times 10^9$/l | $30 \times 10^9$/l |

A variety of etiologic factors have been associated with hematopoietic disease. Disease can be caused by ionizing radiation and also by cytotoxic chemotherapy (alkylating agents and epipodophyllotoxins), although there is scant evidence to suggest that the two together have a synergistic effect. Some industrial chemicals such as benzene are implicated in acute myeloblastic leukemia. A genetic etiologic factor in leukemia has also been suggested. People with Down syndrome have a higher risk of leukemia, and approximately 90% of chronic myeloid leukemia cases are associated with the Philadelphia chromosome (resulting from a translocation between chromosomes 9 and 22). Furthermore, the Epstein–Barr virus (EBV) has been associated with hematopoietic disease of the lymphoid series.

Acute and chronic hematopoietic disease, having been further subdivided by their differentiation pathways (lymphoid or myeloid), can be grouped together to form four major disease categories:

- acute lymphoblastic leukemia (ALL)
- acute myeloblastic leukemia
- chronic lymphocytic leukemia (CLL)
- chronic myelogenous (or myeloid, or granulocytic) leukemia (CML).

Myeloid leukemias may sometimes be referred to as granulocytic or myelocytic. Lymphoid leukemias may be further subdivided into T and B cell types. Note that the terminology used here describes where the malignant cell is on the differentiation pathway. For example, myelo*blastic* indicates that the malignant cell is an immature myelocyte at the beginning of the differentiation pathway. Lympho*cytic* indicates that the malignant cell is a mature lymphocyte toward the end of the differentiation pathway.

## MYELOID DISEASE

Myeloid neoplasms consist of diseases that are commonly considered together because of their origin from the same initial differentiation pathway (see Fig. 2.2). These diseases manifest themselves in overproduction of any one of the resultant blood cells—red cells, platelets, monocytes, basophils, eosinophils, or neutrophils—at the expense of other blood cells.

True malignant hematopoietic disease is sometimes preceded by a group of disorders known as *myelodysplastic syndromes* (MDS), a group of diseases in which the production of blood cells is severely disrupted. Myelodysplasia suggests a problem with the bone marrow, but—in contrast to leukemia, where only one type of blood cell is overproduced—MDS manifests itself in the overproduction of more than one kind, and sometimes all kinds, of blood cells. There are five main varieties of MDS:

- *Refractory anemia* (RA)—Red cells appear abnormal, as may the white and platelet cells. RA accounts for less than one third of all MDS and rarely progresses to acute leukemia.
- *Refractory anemia with ringed sideroblasts* (RAS or RARS)— Same changes as in RA but red cells are more defective in that they are unable to utilize iron for oxygen transportation around the body. The iron forms characteristic rings in the cytoplasm of the red blood cell. The cell is termed a ringed sideroblast. RAS accounts for 2–5% of MDS patients.
- *Refractory anemia with excess blasts* (RAEB)—Along with the abnormal red cells, there is progressive mutation of the white cells and platelets, with increasing abnormal production. RAEB accounts for approximately one third of MDS, and about 40% of cases will progress to acute leukemia.
- *Refractory anemia with excess blasts in transformation* (RAEB-t)—Very similar in features to acute leukemia, the only distinction being the number of blast (immature) cells in the bone marrow. This disease accounts for approximately one quarter of MDS cases, and over 60% of these will progress to acute leukemia.
- *Chronic myelomonocytic leukemia* (CMML)—Red cell precursors appear abnormal and there is an increase in the number of monocytes. As it is a chronic disease, the cells are generally more mature, but the marrow may contain an increased proportion of blast cells. This disease comes under the title of MDS because of the similar blood picture and accounts for approximately one quarter of cases. Around 30% will progress to acute leukemia.

Because of the poor quality of blood cells produced in MDS, many are destroyed prior to entering the circulation and as a result patients often suffer from pancytopenia (decreases in the number of all blood cells) and associated symptoms (see Table 2.4)

MDS is sometimes referred to as pre-leukemia, a term that indicates the possibility that this disease will progress to acute

**Table 2.4**  Some signs and symptoms resulting from underproduction of blood cells

| Blood cell | Symptom if deficient |
| --- | --- |
| Red | Anemia, tiredness, lethargy |
| Platelet | Epistaxis, hematemesis, hematuria, melena, bruising, petechiae |
| Neutrophil | Fever, infection, ulceration, bone pain, lymphadenopathy, hepatomegaly, splenomegaly |

leukemia. Management of these patients is mainly supportive, and attempts to relieve symptoms rather than attempt a cure. In most cases, the disease is treatable but unfortunately not curable; many patients over 50 years of age are ineligible for bone marrow transplant (BMT).

The progression of MDS leads to a group of malignant myeloid diseases. These can also occur spontaneously and can be broadly divided into chronic and acute disease.

The chronic forms of the disease are referred to as *myeloproliferative disorders* and manifest themselves in overproduction of more mature cells from the myeloid series, which may include white or red cells and platelets. The main categories of disease include:

- CML (or myeloid, or granulocytic)
- chronic neutrophilic leukemia
- chronic eosinophilic leukemia
- chronic idiopathic myelofibrosis
- polycythemia vera
- essential thrombocythemia.

All of these diseases may convert into acute myelogenous leukemia, and treatment tends to be of a palliative nature, to relieve symptoms such as splenomegaly and hepatomegaly. There are no known causes of myeloproliferative disorders—except for CML, which is associated with a specific genetic abnormality: the Philadelphia chromosome.

## CML

A disease affecting people around 60 years of age, CML (or myeloid, or granulocytic leukemia) is of particular interest to oncologists, as it is associated with a specific genetic abnormality.

In approximately 95% of cases, the leukemic cells display a chromosomal abnormality associated with a translocation of cytogenetic material between the long arms of chromosomes 9 and 22. The resultant chromosome is called the Philadelphia chromosome. The onset of the disease is slow, as the disease progresses through a chronic phase. The patient usually experiences severe splenomegaly and a significantly elevated white cell count. Thrombocytopenia may also be a presenting symptom. The chronic phase of the disease will eventually transform into an accelerated and subsequently blastic phase, which is typified by increased numbers of immature blast cells in the bone marrow. This phase of the disease often leads to death within the first year.

### Treatment

The chronic phase of the disease can only be treated successfully by allogeneic (i.e. from another person) BMT. Interferon alfa has shown some success in increasing survival. Once the disease has transformed into the accelerated phase, BMT and chemotherapy offer little chance of cure. The blastic phase of the disease can be treated with drugs similar to those used for the acute leukemias, with 5-azacitidine and mitoxantrone offering up to 20% response rates. Local treatment to the enlarged spleen with radiotherapy may be used.

## AML

The acute hematopoietic malignancy that affects the myeloid series is referred to as AML. This is a rare disease affecting mainly older people. Incidence increases after the age of 35. Rates are slightly higher in males and whites, and although a direct etiology is not known, prior exposure to radiation has been associated with onset of the disease. Also, workers who use benzene and people treated for ALL with alkylating agents and epipodophyllotoxins have an increased risk of AML. Presenting symptoms are similar to those above for ALL, but central nervous system (CNS) infiltration is more rare.

AML is diagnosed by bone marrow aspirate, which identifies more than 20% blast cells. The disease can manifest itself in the abnormal production of cells from the myeloid, erythroid or megakaryocytic cells lines. AML is classified using the WHO classification system (see Table 2.2). Distinction of the various subtypes of AML is important and has significant patient management and prognostic implications.

### Treatment

Treatment for AML is similar to that for ALL, and it is important first to get the patient into remission. This is achieved by a combination of chemotherapy drugs such as cytarabine and daunorubicin, which is successful in approximately 70% of patients. Consolidation therapy is continued for those patients achieving remission, with continued doses of cytarabine-containing regimes. Maintenance chemotherapy is not considered a useful option. The best chance of cure for patients is a BMT, which is offered to patients in whom remission has not been achieved, or those who are at high risk of relapse even though induction of remission was successful.

## LYMPHOID DISEASE

Lymphoid neoplasms can be broadly divided into two main groups: B cell neoplasms and T cell neoplasms. Of these, three subgroups can be identified by their individual characteristics:

- *Lymphocytic leukemia*: a lymphoid neoplasm with bone marrow involvement, accompanied by tumor cells in the peripheral blood. Lymphocytic leukemias may suppress hematopoiesis and may also spread and infiltrate into and enlarge the spleen and liver.
- *Lymphoma*: a proliferating discrete mass that mainly affects the lymphatic system of the body. The subtypes are Hodgkin lymphoma (HL) and non-Hodgkin lymphoma (NHL).
- *Plasma cell neoplasms*: mature B cells that are made in the marrow attack bone or soft tissues; also called multiple myeloma.

Bone marrow, and perhaps nodal, biopsies are critical for correct diagnosis of lymphoid neoplasms. Most lymphoid neoplasms are of B cell origin and tend to be associated with immune response deprivation.

## Lymphocytic leukemia

The term lymphocytic leukemia describes neoplasms that manifest in the bone marrow, and this differentiates this type of disease from lymphomas, which present as a disease of the lymphatic system. Lymphocytic leukemia can be subcategorized as acute or chronic and may be of B cell or T cell origin.

## ALL in children

This disease affects mainly children and is the most common form of cancer in childhood. It normally presents between 2 and 8 years of age, with peak incidence at 4 years. There is a slightly higher incidence among boys. Most symptoms are due to infiltration of the bone marrow, causing anemia, thrombocytopenia, bone pain, and infection. Enlargement of lymph nodes, splenomegaly, and hepatomegaly may also be present. Rarely, the patient may present with involvement of the CNS meninges, which may cause headaches and vomiting.

Diagnostic investigation may include bone marrow aspiration and full (complete) blood count. The aim is to detect increased levels of lymphoblasts. Normally, an elevated white blood count is seen, but this may not always be the case. ALL can be classified using the WHO classification (see Table 2.2).

ALL blast cells are derived from either B cell or T cell lineage. B cell leukemias can be further subdivided into four main categories (precursor-B, pre-B, immature, and mature B cell leukemia), according to the degree of differentiation of the cells. Generally, the earlier in the B cell lineage, the younger the patient and the better the prognosis. T cell leukemia can be divided into pre-T cell leukemia and T cell leukemia. These patients tend to be male and older than other ALL patients, and they often present with an enlarged thymus gland (diagnosed on X-ray) and lymphadenopathy.

**Treatment**    Treatment of childhood ALL consists of four phases that may take as long as 2–3 years to complete. Phase one involves inducing remission of the disease. The aim is to get the peripheral blood cell counts to return to near normal. This involves intensive chemotherapy, usually a combination of vincristine, prednisone and L-asparaginase. Induction will be successful in 95% of patients. Phase two involves treatment of the CNS, as this is often a sanctuary site (hiding place where treatment is ineffective) for leukemic cells. Cranial irradiation (18 Gy) and intrathecal methotrexate are the norm. Phase three is one of consolidation/intensification.

High or intermediate doses of methotrexate or other drugs similar to those used to achieve remission may be used during consolidation. Phase four is maintenance, which usually consists of oral 6-mercaptopurine and oral methotrexate for up to 3 years after remission. In boys, there is a chance of relapse in the testes, another leukemic sanctuary site. This can be confirmed at biopsy and the affected testis removed. Testicular radiation may also be administered.

### ALL in adults

The clinical presentation of adult patients is similar to that described above, but a higher proportion will present with a mediastinal mass. About 30% of cases are Philadelphia chromosome positive (Ph+), and this is usually associated with poorer prognosis. Morphologically, the disease is classified similarly to that for childhood ALL. The treatment of adult ALL is similar to the treatment of childhood ALL, although the chemotherapy regimens at remission and consolidation stages may be more intense. Cranial irradiation and intrathecal methotrexate are used to treat the cerebrospinal axis, and testicular relapse is uncommon.

### CLL

CLL is rare in patients younger than 40 years of age and is slightly more common in males. The onset of the disease is insidious; approximately 25% of patients are diagnosed incidentally on routine blood tests or medical examination. Common symptoms include anemia and enlargement of lymph nodes. The spleen may also be enlarged, although not to the same extent as in CML. Elevated white cell counts in the order of $200–300 \times 10^9/l$ is common. Often this disease is grouped together with low grade non-Hodgkin small lymphocytic lymphoma, as it is now recognized that the B lymphocyte is the malignant cell and only the background tissue (bone marrow in leukemia versus lymph nodes in lymphoma) is different.

**Treatment**   There is no known treatment that can cure this disease. However, patients can often live for many years with no therapy.

## Lymphomas

*Oncology*

Lymphomas can occur anywhere in the body where there is lymphatic tissue. The two main types of lymphoma are HL and NHL. HL mainly affects the lymph nodes, and non-Hodgkin lymphoma can affect the diffuse lymphatic tissues throughout the body, although lymph node involvement may occur also.

*HL*

With conventional therapies, Hodgkin lymphoma is now highly curable. A better understanding of how the lymphatic system functions and better staging techniques, along with a greater understanding of how radiotherapy and chemotherapy work, have resulted in considerable success in the management of patients with this type of lymphoma.

The incidence of HL is bimodal. It is rare to develop the disease below 5 years of age. There is a major peak around 15–25 years and a further peak in middle age. HL is slightly more common in males. Although a direct etiologic link is unknown, the majority of cases are associated with the EBV. The disease is characterized by the presence of atypical, multinucleated Reed–Sternberg cells (Fig. 2.4), which replace normal lymphocytes in the lymphatic tissue.

On presentation, patients generally have enlarged lymph nodes in the cervical region, axilla, or supraclavicular regions. This adenopathy differs from the enlargement of normal nodes as a

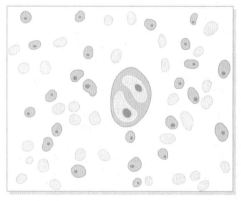

**Figure 2.4** A Reed–Sternberg cell (centre). Note the large, prominent nucleoli.

result of infection, in that the nodes appear more rubbery and firm in HL. The Rye classification has been used since the 1960s to aid microscopic evaluation of the various types of HL. In the late 1980s, a new type of HL was identified as having a distinctly different prognosis. Together, the histologies of the Rye classification (now called classic HL) and nodular lymphocyte predominance comprise the HL cell types of the WHO classification (see Table 2.2). However, because of successful multiagent chemotherapy regimens, histological subtype tends not to influence outcome for patients with HL.

**Staging**   The spread of HL follows the route of the lymphatics from where the disease originated. It is rare for HL to skip lymph node stations. Therefore, knowledge of the lymphatic drainage for areas of the body is crucial in understanding the likely spread of HL. The favored staging system is the Ann Arbor staging system (see Table 2.5). Accurate staging of the disease influences the treatment of patients with HL.

Stages I, II, III, and IV HL are subclassified into A and B categories and subcategories E or S. The E subscript represents extranodal involvement and the S subscript represents involvement of the spleen. In terms of symptoms, A is used for those patients who are asymptomatic and B is used for those patients with any of the following specific symptoms:

- unexplained weight loss (more than 10% of body weight)
- unexplained fever for more than 3 days
- drenching night sweats.

**Table 2.5**   Ann Arbor staging for HL

| Stage | Description |
|---|---|
| I | Involvement of a single lymph region (I) or a single extralymphatic organ ($I_E$) |
| II | Involvement of two or more lymph node regions on the same side of the diaphragm (II) or localized involvement of an extralymphatic organ or site and of one or more lymph node regions on the same side of the diaphragm ($II_E$) |
| III | Involvement of lymph node regions on both sides of the diaphragm (III) which may also be accompanied by localized involvement of an extralymphatic organ or site ($III_E$) or by involvement of the spleen ($III_S$) or both ($III_{ES}$) |
| IV | Diffuse or disseminated involvement of one or more extralymphatic organs or tissues with or without associated lymph node enlargement |

The presence of B symptoms may indicate that the patient has systemic disease even though it may not be evident from clinical staging. Patients with B symptoms are treated with systemic chemotherapy rather than localized radiotherapy.

Stage IV may be further annotated with the following in order to define the extralymphatic organ involved: L, lung; M, bone marrow; O, osseous; P, pleura; H, hepatic; D, derma; S, spleen.

**Treatment**  Modern treatment for HL has led to long-term cure in the majority of patients. The treatment can be summarized as shown in Table 2.6.

Radiotherapy uses mantle or inverted-Y techniques, depending upon whether disease is above or below the diaphragm, respectively, to treat all lymphatic drainage areas associated with the primary tumor. Combination chemotherapy may be MOPP (mustine, Oncovin [vincristine], procarbazine, prednisone), ABVD (Adriamycin [doxorubicin], bleomycin, vinblastine, DTIC), or another combination. In some circumstances, vinblastine may be substituted for vincristine for the combination MVPP.

### NHL

NHL is a general term used to describe a heterogeneous group of malignant disorders that mainly occur in older age groups. Presenting symptoms may be similar to those of HL, although it is more likely that disease involves extranodal or extralymphatic sites. The patient often presents with already disseminated disease and B symptoms. Although the etiology of NHL is unknown, the risk of a person developing NHL is increased in immunodeficiency disorders. Reed–Sternberg cells are not present in NHL. Certain NHLs, such as Burkitt lymphoma, are associated with EBV, especially in African children, in whom the disease is quite common. NHL is an overproliferation of B cells or T cells—lymphocytes that have different differentiation pathways—thus, there are many

**Table 2.6**  Summary of treatment of HL

| Stage | Treatment |
|---|---|
| IA, IIA | Radiotherapy |
| IIA (bulky mediastinum) | Radiotherapy and chemotherapy |
| IB, IIB, IIIA, IIIB, IVA, IVB | Chemotherapy |

forms and names of lymphoma. T cells are formed and migrate to the thymus in fetal life. They differentiate into a range of T cells with differing functions, including helper T cells, suppressor T cells, memory T cells, and killer T cells. These then migrate to lymph nodes and lodge in the paracortical region of the lymph node. B cells are formed in the fetal liver and migrate to the bone marrow, and from there migrate to the lymph nodes where they lodge in the follicle of the lymph node, which contains a germinal center and an outer margin. These T and B cell derivations form the basis of the WHO classification for all lymphoid neoplasms (Table 2.2). The majority of NHLs are from the B cell series.

**Staging**    The staging system for NHL is similar to that for HL, the Ann Arbor. Non-contiguous lymph node involvement, which is uncommon in HL, is more common among patients with NHL. Extralymphatic involvement of the gastrointestinal tract, brain, uterus, and breast is also more common. A single extranodal or extralymphatic site is occasionally the only site of involvement in

**Table 2.7**  General principles in the management of NHL

| Extent of disease | Management |
| --- | --- |
| Early stage, localized | Radiotherapy is the mainstay of treatment |
| Late stage, diffuse | Slow-growing tumor is very difficult to treat, as conventional radiotherapy and chemotherapy are not curative. Treatment may be deferred until the patient becomes symptomatic. If treatment is considered, single agent chemotherapy may be an option |
| Aggressive early stage | Combination chemotherapy, with or without radiotherapy |
| Aggressive late stage | Combination chemotherapy, with radiotherapy for bulky disease; may consider bone marrow transplant |
| Highly aggressive NHL | Burkitt lymphoma and lymphoblastic lymphoma are treated with aggressive combination chemotherapy and CNS prophylactic treatment because of the likelihood of cranial tumor deposits/recurrence. Treatment is similar to that given for ALL |
| Gastric NHL | A disease associated with *Helicobacter pylori* bacteria. Treatment with appropriate antibiotics may reduce and even cure the tumor. On recurrence, local radiotherapy, chemotherapy, and/or surgery are options |

Early stage includes Ann Arbor stages I and II; late stage includes Ann Arbor stages III and IV.

patients with diffuse lymphoma. Bone marrow and hepatic involvement are especially common in patients with low grade lymphomas, and cytological examination of cerebrospinal fluid (CSF) may be positive in patients with aggressive NHL.

**Treatment**    The treatment of NHL depends in large part on the histological type, location, and stage of the disease. However, some general principles can be applied (see Table 2.7).

## SELF-ASSESSMENT QUESTIONS

Answer true or false to the following. Answers are on page 243.

1. The circulatory system is synonymous with the cardiovascular system.
2. The blood cells make up most of the plasma in blood.
3. Red bone marrow is a rich source of blood-producing tissue.
4. Pluripotential means that the cell is able to become different types of cell.
5. Hematopoietic stem cells can follow the myeloid or lymphoid pathways of differentiation.
6. Platelets are otherwise referred to as basophils.
7. Lymph drains towards organs and tissues.
8. Ultimately, the lymphatic vessels join with the blood circulation.
9. Lymph nodes contain lymphocytes.
10. Hematopoietic disease manifests in an overproduction of one or more types of blood cell.
11. Chronic hematopoietic disease is typified by the presence of primitive blast cells in the bone marrow and peripheral blood.
12. Myeloid disease results in an overproduction of T lymphocytes.
13. Refractory anemia (with ringed sideroblasts) accounts for the majority of myelodysplastic syndromes.
14. Pancytopenia refers to abnormally low numbers of all types of blood cell.
15. Myeloproliferative disorders manifest themselves in over-production of the more mature cells from the myeloid series.
16. Chronic myeloid leukemia is associated with the Philadelphia chromosome.
17. Acute myeloid leukemia is diagnosed by bone marrow aspirate that contains more than 50% blast cells.
18. Acute lymphoblastic leukemia mainly affects adults.
19. Chronic lymphocytic leukemia and non-Hodgkin small lymphocytic lymphoma are recognized by the World Health Organization as the same type of disease.
20. Hodgkin lymphoma is typified by the presence of Reed–Sternberg cells.

# The connective tissues

Connective tissue is the packaging material of the body: separating, protecting, and supporting various organs. All the cells of the connective system arise from a layer of tissue found in the early embryo called the mesoderm, the cells of which are called mesenchyme cells (see Ch. 1). This middle layer of the developing embryo differentiates into all types of connective tissues, including cartilage, bone, and the connective tissue proper, as well as muscle, blood, and the vessels of the blood and lymphatic systems. Figure 3.1 shows the differentiation pathways from a mesenchyme cell to the cells of various connective tissues. This shared origin is perhaps why their oncology and forms of treatment are similar. Each type of connective tissue originates from an immature type of cell called a blast cell. Blast cells continually reproduce themselves and are found in fibrous tissue (fibroblasts), in cartilage (chondroblasts), and in bone (osteoblasts). They all produce a matrix that consists of a fluid, semi-fluid, gelatinous, or calcified ground substance and protein fibers, the consistency of which depends on the type of cell that produces it. Once the matrix is secreted, the blast cells differentiate into mature cells, which are then known as fibrocytes, chondrocytes, and osteocytes, respectively.

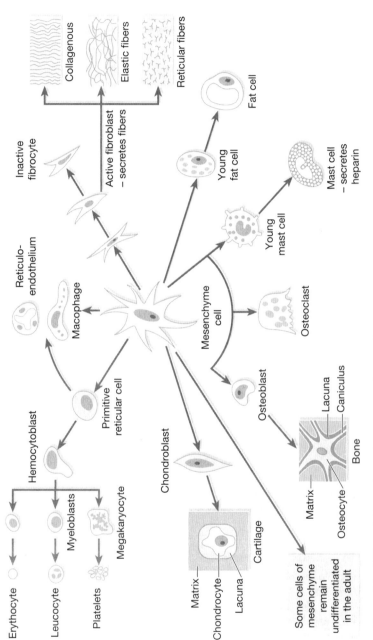

**Figure 3.1** Differentiation pathways from a mesenchyme cell to mature connective tissues.

## TYPES OF CONNECTIVE TISSUE
### Cartilage

Cartilage can also be divided into three main types: hyaline cartilage, fibrocartilage, and elastic cartilage (Fig. 3.2a).

  • Hyaline cartilage is an elastic tissue with a firm matrix, filled
with groups of cells called chondrocytes, which lie in the lacunae.
Hyaline cartilage is an earlier, more immature form of bone and is
found as the costal cartilage in ribs, trachea, larynx, and bronchi.
Hyaline cartilage is also found on the articular surfaces of some
bones, at synovial joints.

  • Fibrocartilage forms a tissue with a mass of white fibers as
the matrix, with many fewer chondrocytes than hyaline cartilage.
Fibrocartilage is still a strong tissue but has much more elasticity
than the hyaline type. It is found in areas of the body that need
extra cushioning and protection, such as the disks between vertebrae in the spine.

  • Elastic cartilage is a mass of yellow fibers in a matrix with very
few chondrocytes; this tissue is found in the pinna (external part
of the ear) and epiglottis.

### Bone

Bone is one of the hardest tissues of the body and forms the skeleton, which is made up of 206 bones in the adult. The skeleton
is the framework of the human body, to which all other organs
and tissues are attached. The skeleton is divided into two parts:
the axial skeleton, composed of the skull, spine, and ribs; and
the appendicular skeleton (Latin *appendere*: to hang onto), which
includes bones of the upper and lower limbs (extremities) plus the
shoulder girdle and pelvic girdle.

Bone is covered by a protective, fibrous membrane called the
periosteum (see Fig. 3.3). The periosteum is composed of two layers: an outer tough fibrous layer which gives strength, and an inner
thinner layer that provides nourishment via a blood supply and has
specialized bone cells called osteoblasts. Osteoblasts are stimulated
to produce a protective cuff around a break so repair can occur from
within the bone. Under the periosteum are two further layers: an
outer layer of hard, compact bone, which provides the supportive
strength of the bone and in long bones forms the major part of the
shaft (or diaphysis) (see Fig. 3.3); and an inner layer of cancellous

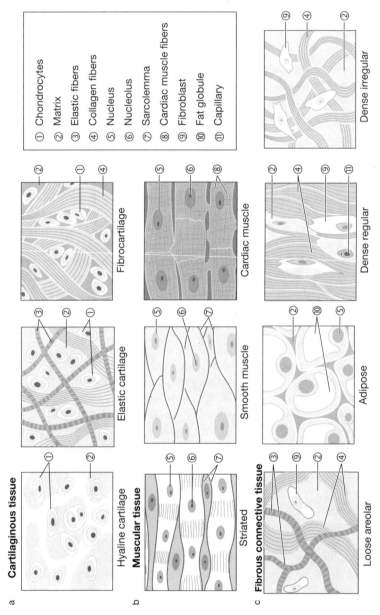

**Figure 3.2** Mature connective tissue: (a) cartilaginous; (b) muscular; (c) fibrous connective tissue.

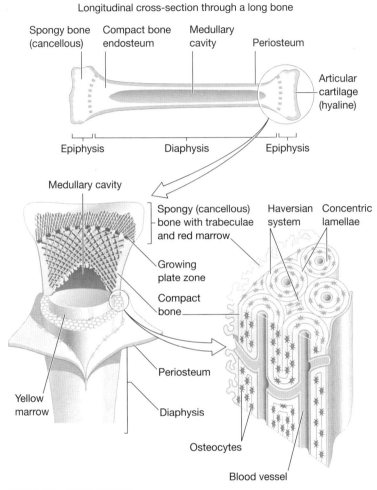

Longitudinal cross-section through a long bone

Figure 3.3   Bone structure.

or spongy bone. Compact bone is made up of closely packed units called osteons or the Haversian system. The osteon is made up of concentric layers called lamellae with spaces between layers, called lacunae. In these lacunae lie the bone cells or osteocytes. Cancellous or spongy bone is made of a network whose parts are called trabeculae, and which gives lightness and strength to the bone. The trabeculae provide spaces for red bone marrow and are found at the epiphyses (growth ends) of long bones and in other bones which do not have a medullary cavity (the central space in long bones which is filled with marrow). In a young child the medullary cavity is full of red marrow, a thick jelly-like substance responsible for blood cell production, and is full of red and white blood cells all at different stages of development. As the child matures, this red marrow gradually changes into yellow marrow which no longer produces blood cells. By adulthood the areas of blood-producing marrow are reduced to the head of the femur, the head of the humerus, the flat bones, and the irregular hipbone. The latter two are common sites for bone marrow biopsy. The proportion of compact to spongy bone varies with different types of bones, which can be classified according to their shape—long, short, flat, and irregular.

Bone has a number of important roles:

- support
- protection
- 'store' for minerals—calcium and phosphate are released as ions into the bloodstream and later returned to bone; an imbalance in this exchange can exacerbate the condition of osteoporosis in later life
- blood cell formation site—hematopoiesis occurs in the red marrow of certain bones.

## Muscle

There are three main types of muscle tissue: striated muscle, smooth muscle, and cardiac muscle (see Fig. 3.2b).

*Striated muscle (rhabdomyo-)* is under voluntary control. It allows movement, as in the extension and flexion of the upper arm by the presence of two sets of opposing muscle groups: the biceps brachii and triceps. Striated muscle tissue is so called because its appearance under a microscope is of bands of alternating dark and light stripes. Striated muscle cells are cylindrical in shape; there can be more than one nucleus in each cell and their length can vary from a few millimeters to over 30 centimeters. For example, striated muscles can range from small muscles in the front of the neck (suprahyoid and infrahyoid), which aid the act of swallowing, to the sartorius muscle, the longest muscle in the body, arising in the pelvis and attached to the medial surface of the tibia of the lower leg. A protective layer called the sarcolemma covers the muscle cell. Striated muscle cells are grouped into bundles and covered by strong white connective tissue called the muscle fascia. Striated muscle is found mainly on the appendicular skeleton.

*Smooth muscle (leiomyo-)* or involuntary muscle is found in the walls of the gastrointestinal tract, ureters, bladder, and blood and lymphatic vessels. These cells are spindle shaped and have one central nucleus. They also form bundles, but they are held together by sheets of areolar tissue.

*Cardiac muscle* is only found in the heart and is unique in its power of sustained rhythmic contractions.

## GENERAL ONCOLOGY OF CONNECTIVE TISSUE

Sarcoma is the term generally used to describe a malignant tumor in connective tissue. However, benign tumors of soft tissue (non-bone connective tissue) are much more common than malignant ones. Benign and malignant tumors of connective tissue are listed in Table 3.1.

Soft tissue sarcomas can occur in any part of the body, in any connective tissue—muscle, fat, fibrous tissue, and blood vessels—and at any age. In adults sarcomas tend to occur in middle to later years. In children, soft tissue sarcomas are the fourth most common malignancy in the UK, and account for about 7% of all pediatric malignancies. The most common type in children is

**Table 3.1**  Types of connective tissue and associated benign and malignant tumors

| Connective tissue type | Sites found | Benign tumor (-oma) | Malignant tumor (-sarcoma) |
| --- | --- | --- | --- |
| Cartilage | Long bones around knees, pelvis, and hand joints | Chondroma | Chondrosarcoma |
| Bone | Long bones around knee, shoulder, wrist | Osteoma | Osteosarcoma, Ewing's sarcoma |
| Fat | Surface of shoulders, buttocks, deep in muscles, between the spine and intestine (retroperitoneum) | Lipoma | Liposarcoma |
| Fibrous tissue | Skin, bone, ovary, breast | Fibroma | Fibrosarcoma |
| Voluntary muscle | Muscles of appendicular skeleton (arms, legs, etc.) | Rhabdomyoma (rare) | Rhabdomyosarcoma |
| Involuntary muscle | Skin, stomach, intestines | Leiomyoma | Leiomyosarcoma |

rhabdomyosarcoma, which develops from striated muscle. It is most often found in the head and neck region and genitourinary system. Most soft tissue sarcomas occur spontaneously, and those that do not are often associated with a genetic mutation. Exposure to radiation can increase the risk of developing sarcomas, and children are especially at risk. Sarcomas tend to occur in a younger age group than do carcinomas.

## Presenting symptoms

Patients usually see the doctor because of a painless lump that could have been present for weeks or months. The tumor invades local soft tissue, nerves, and blood vessels, which leads to early blood-borne spread to the lungs. Lymphatic involvement is uncommon except in the case of synovial sarcoma and alveolar rhabdomyosarcoma. Retroperitoneal sarcomas can grow to a considerable size before giving symptoms, the most common being backache, and movement can become limited if the sarcoma is close to joints.

## Staging

The staging of soft tissue sarcomas is the most important indicator to determine appropriate treatment. Box 3.1 and Table 3.2 show the TNM definitions and stage groups for all sarcomas except those of bone and cartilage. The latest American Joint Committee on Cancer (AJCC)/Union Internationale Contre Le Cancer (IUCC) TNM classification recommends that grades be assigned to all sarcomas; previously there were a number of different grading systems which have varied in grade groupings or number of tiers (a three-tiered and, less commonly, a four-tiered system). As clinicians prefer a two-tiered system (low versus high) for recording data, the new recommendations accommodate this by translating the three- and four-tiered grades into a two-tiered system.

## Treatment

Patients with an early stage (stage I) soft tissue sarcoma may be treated with surgery alone if the tumor can be completely resected, including a wide margin of normal tissue. This leaves the patient with a good functional and cosmetic result. However, at later stages (stage II), radiotherapy is administered before

**Box 3.1** Definition of TNM symbols used in staging all sarcomas except those of bone and cartilage.

**Primary tumor**
- TX: Primary tumor cannot be assessed
- T0: No evidence of primary tumor
- T1: Tumor 5 cm or less in greatest dimension
  —T1a: Superficial tumor—located exclusively above the superficial fascia without invasion of the fascia
  —T1b: Deep tumor—located exclusively beneath the superficial fascia, or superficial to the fascia with invasion of or through the fascia, or both superficial yet beneath the fascia. (Retroperitoneal, mediastinal, and pelvic sarcomas are classified as deep tumors.)
- T2: Tumor more than 5 cm in greatest dimension
  —T2a: Superficial tumor (as defined above)
  —T2b: Deep tumor (as defined above)

**Regional node involvement**
- NX: Regional lymph nodes cannot be assessed
- N0: No regional lymph node metastasis
- N1: Regional lymph node metastasis

**Distant metastasis**
- MX: Distant metastasis cannot be assessed
- M0: No distant metastasis
- M1: Distant metastasis

**Table 3.2** Summary of stage grouping for all sarcomas except those of bone and cartilage: four stages defined according to three different grading systems

| Stage | Primary tumor | Regional node involvement | Distant metastasis | Grading system | | |
|---|---|---|---|---|---|---|
| | | | | Four-tier | Three-tier | Two-tier[a] |
| I | T1a, T1b, T2a, or T2b | N0 | M0 | G1–2 | G1 | Low |
| II | T1a, T1b, or T2a | N0 | M0 | G3–4 | G2–3 | High |
| III | T2b | N0 | M0 | G3–4 | G2–3 | High |
| IV | Any T | N1 | M0 | Any G | Any G | High or low |
| | Any T | N0 | M1 | Any G | Any G | High or low |

[a] Recommended in *TNM Classification of Malignant Tumours*, 6th edn.

surgery, as the tumor is more likely to recur locally. Incomplete excision may be supplemented by radiotherapy. Combination chemotherapy is often used, and doxorubicin (Adriamycin) is the most commonly used agent. At stages II and III, a number of patients will have tumors that recur, and although chemotherapy can increase the disease-free interval, it has not affected patients' overall survival.

## Prognosis

Patients with early stage disease have a very good prognosis. Unfortunately, in later stages the outlook is much poorer, with approximately only half the patients disease-free at 5 years.

## OSTEOSARCOMA

Osteosarcoma is the most common primary malignant tumor of bone. It arises in the bone-forming cells called osteoblasts. There are two peak age ranges: the first peak appears in adolescence (three quarters of patients are in this group) between the ages of 10 and 20 years, accounting for about 5% of childhood and adolescent tumors; the second peak appears in the elderly (over 60s), often due to a complication of Paget's disease or of previous radiotherapy. Osteosarcoma is slightly more common in males and typically arises in the metaphyses of long bones, such as the distal femur. In children, over 50% of osteosarcomas arise in the proximal tibia or proximal femur. In the older patient, osteosarcoma can arise in flat as well as long bones. As the tumor enlarges it produces osteoid tissue, forces through the cortex, and raises the periosteum. This gives rise to the classic appearance seen on X-ray called Codman's triangle. 'Skip' lesions may also occur where tumor cells may not invade immediately adjacent normal tissue, but then invade normal tissue some distance away from the primary tumor. It is vital that treatment must take this into account, as it will lead to local recurrence.

## Etiology

There is no known cause of osteosarcoma; however, there are a number of genetic mutations which are associated with an increased risk of developing osteosarcomas or sarcomas. Li-Fraumeni syndrome, resulting from a mutation of the *p53* tumor suppressor gene, causes the cell to go out of control, leading to an overproduction of cells and the development of sarcomas before the mid-40s, a relatively early age. An increased frequency of osteosarcoma (up to 400-fold) is associated with families with hereditary retinoblastoma (an *Rb* gene mutation which prevents it from functioning properly as a tumor suppressor gene).

## Presenting symptoms

Often the patient may be asymptomatic, and a pathological fracture through the tumor may be the first indication of any disease. Confusion and delays in treatment can arise as osteosarcoma symptoms can mimic osteomyelitis. Aggressive tumors often cause systemic symptoms, including fever, sweats, and so forth. Osteomyelitis is an infection of the bone characterized by a high fever alternating with chills, pain, nausea, and edema in the affected limb.

## Staging

Although the TNM staging system is gaining wider acceptance (see Box 3.2 and Table 3.3), you may find that osteosarcomas are classified into groups depending on their site of origin:

- central group tumors which derive from the medullary cavity and include:
  —high grade central osteosarcoma (accounting for 70% of all osteosarcomas)
  —telangiectatic osteosarcoma
  —intraosseous low grade osteosarcoma
  —small round cell osteosarcoma
- peripheral group tumors which arise from the surface of the bone and include:
  —parosteal low grade osteosarcoma
  —periosteal osteosarcoma (low–intermediate grade)
  —high grade surface osteosarcoma.

---

**Box 3.2** Definition of TNM symbols used in staging osteosarcomas

**Primary tumor**
- TX: Primary tumor cannot be assessed
- T0: No evidence of primary tumor
- T1: Tumor 8 cm or less in greatest dimension
- T2: Tumor more than 8 cm in greatest dimension
- T3: Discontinuous tumors in the primary bone site

**Regional node involvement**
- NX: Regional lymph nodes cannot be assessed
- N0: No regional lymph node involvement
- N1: Regional lymph node involvement

**Distant metastasis**
- MX: Distant metastasis cannot be assessed
- M0: No distant metastasis
- M1: Distant metastasis
  - —M1a: Lung
  - —M1b: Other distant sites

---

**Table 3.3** Summary of stage grouping for osteosarcoma

| Stage | Primary tumor | Regional node involvement | Distant metastasis | Grading system | |
|-------|---------------|---------------------------|--------------------|----------------|----------|
| | | | | Four-tier | Two-tier |
| IA | T1 | N0 | M0 | G1–2 | Low |
| IB | T2 | N0 | M0 | G1–2 | Low |
| IIA | T1 | N0 | M0 | G3–4 | High |
| IIB | T2 | N0 | M0 | G3–4 | High |
| III | T3 | N0 | M0 | Any G | High or low |
| IVA | Any T | N0 | M1a | Any G | High or low |
| IVB | Any T | N1 | Any M | Any G | High or low |
| | Any T | Any N | M1b | Any G | High or low |

# Treatment

The mainstay of treatment for osteosarcoma is surgery, which aims to avoid amputation in favor of limb sparing. Where the resectability of the tumor is the most important prognostic factor, the use of concurrent chemotherapy has greatly improved survival rates, with typical combination regimens that include doxorubicin and cisplatin. Preoperative chemotherapy has been useful to reduce tumor size and has allowed previously unsuitable patients to have surgery, and this has increased overall survival rates. Because of the radioresistant nature of osteosarcoma, high doses are required to be effective, so radiotherapy is reserved for tumors difficult to fully resect or where it is felt that micrometastases may be left behind.

## Prognosis

With the use of concurrent chemotherapy, overall survival rates of 50–80% can be achieved. Unfortunately, up to 20% of patients already have metastases at the time of diagnosis. However, with aggressive chemotherapy, up to 40% of these patients have the chance of long-term survival.

## EWING'S SARCOMA

Ewing's sarcoma accounts for about 60% of cases of a group of tumors which all derive from the same primordial stem cell or tissue formed in the early stages of embryonic development. This group also includes extraosseous Ewing's sarcoma (very rare) and primitive neuroectodermal tumors (sometimes called PNET or peripheral neuroepithelioma). Ewing's sarcoma is a primary malignant bone tumor that mainly affects children and adolescents, particularly between the ages of 10 and 16 years, and often coincides with periods of rapid bone growth, yet Ewing's sarcoma remains rare in all groups of the population. At the time of diagnosis, most patients with Ewing's sarcomas display a change in genetic make-up. A piece of chromosome 11 moves to chromosome 22 and vice versa—a *translocation*, t(11;22), where the combination of two unrelated genes creates a new gene which seems to be involved with abnormal control of other genes. This t(11;22) translocation is unique to Ewing's and other PNET tumors. This genetic change only occurs in the tumor cells, so it is not passed from parent to child, or from patients to their progeny. It accounts for 4% of childhood malignancies and affects slightly more males than females; it is rare in black populations. Ewing's sarcoma can arise anywhere in the appendicular skeleton, but the commonest sites are the proximal humerus, femur and pelvis. Ewing's sarcoma typically arises at the diaphysis of the bone, growing subperiosteally; as the tumor enlarges and lays down further bone cells, it can give rise to an 'onion skin' appearance which can be seen on X-ray. The symptoms

**Table 3.4** Prognostic indicators in Ewing's sarcoma

| Prognostic indicator | Risk factors | Relative effect on prognosis |
|---|---|---|
| Site of tumor | Pelvis, ribs, and proximal extremities | Unfavorable |
| Size of tumor | Larger than about 10 cm | Unfavorable |
| Sex | Female | Favorable |
| Age | Younger child | Favorable |
| Chemotherapy | Good response to induction course | Favorable |
| Metastases | Present | Unfavorable |

are very similar to those of other sarcomas and only differ in their sporadic nature; Ewing's sarcoma can cause extreme pain.

## Treatment

Chemotherapy is the mainstay of treatment, and has improved the outlook for patients with Ewing's sarcoma and peripheral neuro-ectodermal tumors substantially. Over 90% of patients already have micrometastases even though the primary appears localized at the time of diagnosis, and the micrometastases may be undetected by diagnostic tests. Chemotherapy is given before and after local treatment—which often is surgical resection if the tumor is easily accessible (located in the extremities)—and this produces better functional and cosmetic results. Radiotherapy is only used as treatment for unresectable tumors, as radiation stunts growth and is known to induce secondary tumors in later life. High doses of 40–60 Gy with concurrent chemotherapy give good local control.

## Prognosis

The outlook for patients was very poor until chemotherapy trials in the late 1980s established effective regimens; now, because of these, more than 50% of patients with localized disease are disease-free at 5 years. However, if metastases are present, the 5-year survival drops to 20–30%. Prognostic indicators are summarized in Table 3.4.

## CHONDROSARCOMA

Chondrosarcoma is a malignant tumor of cartilage and is the second most common bone tumor after osteosarcoma. Males are twice as likely to develop chondrosarcoma as females, and it rarely develops before the age of 30. The most common sites are the shoulder, pelvis, and ribs. There is no known cause; however, there is an association with Paget's disease and pre-existing bone disease such as osteochondromas, especially enchondromata (a benign cartilage tumor that, as it grows, stays confined within the metaphysis of long bones). Usually slow-growing, it gives rise to a painful enlarging mass with a wide range of malignancies that are graded from G1 through G4. The majority of tumors are well differentiated with a low risk of metastasis.

## Treatment

Surgery is the treatment of choice if the tumor is well to moderately differentiated. If the tumor is completely resected the prognosis is good, and the majority of these tumors tend to be of low grade. The higher grades are more aggressive, and chemotherapy must be started early. If the tumor is unresectable, radiotherapy may be used.

## Prognosis

Overall, the 5-year survival is approximately 35%. Well to moderately differentiated tumors tend to metastasize very late, if at all. Poorly differentiated tumors tend to metastasize early, and the prognosis is much poorer.

## OSTEOCLASTOMA (GIANT CELL TUMOR)

This is a rare bone tumor, which derives from the large bone-absorbing cells called osteoclasts. Sometimes known as malignant giant cell, this tumor occurs in adults and normally presents between 20 and 40 years of age. It can arise in any bone but most often occurs in long bones, particularly the distal femur or proximal tibia, and up to half arise in the humerus and radius. These tumors demonstrate a classic 'soap bubble' appearance caused by large lytic lesions that are composed of spindle and multinucleate giant cells that expand and eventually destroy the outer bony cortex. Most osteoclastomas are low grade, but there may be late blood-borne metastases to the lungs.

## Treatment

As in other sarcomas, surgery is the treatment of choice. It is essential to obtain clear margins, as the tumor will recur in one third of patients and another third will have a high grade tumor. Overall 5-year survival rate is about 65–70%.

## RHABDOMYOSARCOMA

Rhabdomyosarcoma differs from other soft tissue sarcomas in that, first, 70% of patients are children (the average age is 4 years at the time of diagnosis) and, second, when it metastasizes, the spread is to bone marrow and lymph nodes. Table 3.5 summarizes features of the disease.

### Treatment

All children should receive some chemotherapy and surgery if feasible, and, depending on success of surgery, the addition of radiotherapy should be considered. In order to maximize treatment effect and reduce morbidity, two cycles of chemotherapy are given to patients with a favorable prognosis, and more aggressive regimens are reserved for patients with less favorable histologies.

### Prognosis

Embryonal rhabdomyosarcoma is very curable with current chemotherapy regimens: over 60% of patients are alive and well at 5 years. However, long-term follow-up is required, as long-term effects are now being exhibited by these patients. Alveolar rhabdomyosarcoma has a poorer outlook than embryonal. In adults with embryonal rhabdomyosarcoma, although the tumor responds well to the children's chemotherapy regimens, the overall prognosis is much poorer.

## KAPOSI'S SARCOMA

This is a dermal tumor which appears as purplish-red lesions of the skin. There are four types:

• Classic Kaposi's sarcoma is found in eastern European elderly men, usually on the lower limbs; the disease has a prolonged, slow progress, but will eventually metastasize. This group is also at risk of a second malignancy, non-Hodgkin lymphoma.

**Table 3.5** Features of rhabdomyosarcoma

| Histology | Subtype histologies | Features of tumor | Occurrence | Chromosome translocation | Likely prognosis |
|---|---|---|---|---|---|
| Embryonal (arise in head, neck, and genitourinary) | Botryoidal | Mucosal surfaces of body orifices: vagina, bladder, nares, biliary tract | Majority in childhood | 13 | Good (except if adult) |
| | Spindle | Testes | | | |
| Alveolar | None | In child, extremities; in adolescent, trunk | In children and adults | 13, 2, or 1 | In children not as good as embryonal, but worse if adult |
| Pleomorphic | None | | Majority in adults | Not known | Poor |

- African Kaposi's sarcoma, as the name suggests, is endemic to equatorial Africa. It is mainly a disease of males and tends to occur in younger age groups. The disease has a range of behavior from indolent to very aggressive, where the tumor invades locally.
- Kaposi's sarcoma associated with immunosuppression for organ transplantation. If Kaposi's sarcoma arises, the immunotherapy may have to be delayed or drugs dosage reduced so that the disease may regress.
- Epidemic Kaposi's sarcoma is closely associated with acquired immune deficiency syndrome (AIDS). It presents commonly as a widely spread disease that has very sudden onset and severe effects. There is a strong association with human herpesvirus 8. The incidence of epidemic Kaposi's sarcoma is strongly related to how the disease is acquired. There is a much higher risk of developing Kaposi's sarcoma in homosexual men with human immuno-deficiency virus (HIV) compared with heterosexual men or intravenous drug users with HIV.

## Treatment

Treatment is dependent on how much disease is present. Kaposi's sarcoma is quite radiosensitive; low dose radiotherapy can be administered to a solitary lesion or small groups of lesions and gives good local control. Intravenous chemotherapy may be used, particularly where radiotherapy would be difficult, such as in the oral cavity. If the tumor is widespread, systemic chemotherapy has to be used. Interferon has been quite effective, but if the disease affects visceral organs, or the patient has had repeated infections, interferon is less effective, and single agent or multiple chemotherapy can give reasonable response rates of about 25%.

## Prognosis

The outlook for all patients depends on maintaining local control.

## SELF-ASSESSMENT QUESTIONS

Answer true or false to the following. Answers are on page 243.

1. Every type of connective tissue derives from an immature type of cell called a blast cell.
2. The protective fibrous outer layer of the bone is called the cortex.
3. Chondrocytes are groups of cells found in cartilage.
4. Striated muscle is not under voluntary control.
5. Sarcoma is the term for all types of connective tissue tumors.
6. The most common connective tissue tumor in children is Ewing's sarcoma.
7. The majority of sarcomas arise spontaneously.
8. Sarcomas in general present with a painful lump.
9. Osteosarcoma is the most common primary malignant bone tumor.
10. The classic appearance of osteosarcoma on X-ray is called Codman's triangle.
11. Ewing's sarcoma arises in the appendicular skeleton.
12. In most cases of Ewing's sarcoma there is a specific genetic mutation: the chromosome translocation t(11;22).
13. Surgery is the treatment of choice for Ewing's sarcoma.
14. In chondrosarcoma, the shoulder, pelvis, and ribs are the most common sites.
15. The majority of chondrosarcomas are of low grade and have a low risk of metastasis.
16. In Ewing's sarcoma, the older the child, the better the prognosis.
17. Osteoclastomas have a high risk of recurrence.
18. In rhabdomyosarcoma, 70% of patients are children.
19. Embryonal rhabdomyosarcoma has the best prognosis of the sarcomas.
20. African Kaposi's sarcoma is mainly a disease of elderly men.

# 4

# The nervous system

The nervous system is the control system of the body, carrying out many activities that can be divided into sensory, integrative, and motor functions. We are able to sense external and internal stimuli, interpret the changes sensed, and respond to this change by muscular contraction or glandular secretion. The nervous system, along with the endocrine system, maintains homeostasis within the body; in other words, these two systems keep the internal environment constant.

The various subdivisions of the nervous system can be seen in Figure 4.1, the principal division being between the central nervous

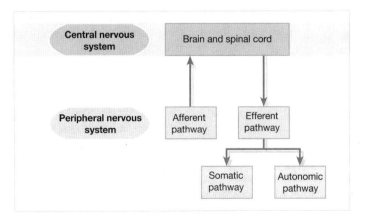

**Figure 4.1**   Subdivisions of the nervous system.

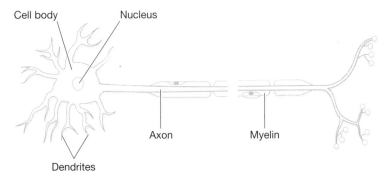

**Figure 4.2** A neuron.

system (CNS) and the peripheral nervous system (PNS). The PNS incorporates an afferent pathway conveying information *to* the CNS and an efferent pathway conveying information *away from* the CNS. Furthermore, the efferent pathway is divided into the somatic and autonomic pathways. The somatic pathway carries nerve impulses to skeletal muscle, which is under conscious control and produces voluntary movement, whereas the autonomic pathway carries impulses to smooth muscle, glands, and cardiac muscle, which are not under conscious control and therefore move involuntarily.

The nervous system consists of only two types of cells: neurons (nerve cells) and neuroglia (glial cells which support the neurons). Neurons are cells that carry messages through the body by electrochemical processes, and they differ from other cells in the body in that they have specialized extensions called dendrites and axons (Fig. 4.2), which bring information to and from the cell body, respectively.

Axons may be covered by a myelin sheath, which insulates the axon and increases nerve impulse speed. Neurons, after about 6 months of age, lose the mitotic apparatus enabling cell division to occur, which means that nerve cells have a limited ability to regenerate and renew themselves. As a result, many are never replaced when they die; consequently, the number of nerve cells is reduced as the body ages. It is rare, therefore, to develop malignant tumors of neurons. The vast majority of malignant tumors of the CNS are of the supporting glial cells.

In the peripheral nervous system, there may be some repair of damage, because different supporting cells are responsible for the

**Table 4.1** Supporting cells of the nervous system

| Cell type | Description | Function | Tumor type |
|---|---|---|---|
| Astrocyte | Star-shaped cells with many projections (astro = star) | Provide neurons with physical and nutritional support; clean up debris; transport nutrients; hold neurons in place; digest parts of dead neurons; and regulate the content of extracellular space | Astrocytoma |
| Oligodendrocytes | Similar to astrocytes but with fewer projections (oligo = few) | Provide insulation; provide support by semi-rigid connective tissue between neurons; and produce myelin sheath around axons of CNS | Oligodendroglioma |
| Microglia | Small cells (micro). Also referred to as brain macrophages because they destroy dead cells and microbes | Digest parts of dead cells and destroy microbes | Microglioma |
| Ependyma | Single layer of epithelial cells; shapes range from squamous to columnar; may be ciliated | Form epithelial lining for ventricles of brain and central canal of spinal cord. Related to circulation of CSF | Ependymoma |
| Schwann cells | Flattened cells | Provide insulation; produce myelin sheath around axons of PNS | Schwannoma (tend to be benign) |

CNS, central nervous system; CSF, cerebrospinal fluid; PNS, peripheral nervous system.

myelination in the two systems. In the PNS, myelination of axons is performed by neurolemmocytes or Schwann cells, which proliferate after damage to the axon. In the CNS, myelination is performed by oligodendrocytes that do not survive after damage to the axon. Myelin gives a white appearance to brain tissue, and unmyelinated axons appear gray; hence the terms white and gray matter when referring to tissues of the CNS.

Glial cells have many important functions without which neurons would not work (see Table 4.1).

## THE CNS

### The brain

The brain is composed of the cerebrum, cerebellum, diencephalon, and brainstem, the lower end of which is continuous with the spinal cord (see Fig. 4.3).

The *cerebrum*, the largest component of the brain, is composed of the right and left cerebral hemispheres. An outer layer of gray matter, the cerebral cortex, is arranged in a number of folds called gyri or convolutions. The deep grooves that occur between these folds are called fissures or sulci, the largest of which, the longitudinal fissure, incompletely separates the two hemispheres. Below

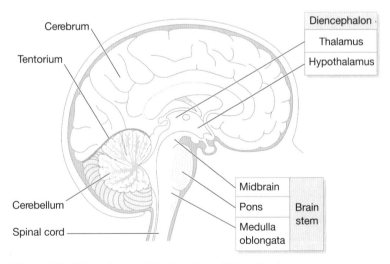

**Figure 4.3** Principal parts of the brain in sagittal section.

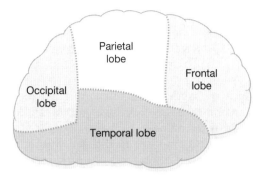

**Figure 4.4** The lobes of the brain.

this fissure the two hemispheres are connected by the corpus cal-
losum, which is a large bundle of nerve fibers. Each hemisphere is
divided descriptively into four lobes (Fig. 4.4)—the frontal, parietal,
temporal, and occipital lobes—which derive their names from the
cranial bones which cover them.

The different areas of the cerebral cortex have different functions
(Table 4.2), which account for varied tumor symptoms, depending on the area involved. Symptoms will also depend on which
side of the brain is involved, as each side appears to be more
important for some functions than others. The right hemisphere is
more important for left hand control, sight, touch, taste, smell and
sound, whereas the left hemisphere is more important for right
hand control, reasoning, language and numerical skills.

The *cerebellum,* the second largest component of the brain, lies
below the occipital lobes of the cerebrum. Like the cerebrum, it
is divided into two hemispheres, each containing different lobes

**Table 4.2** The functions of the lobes of the brain

| Lobe | Function |
| --- | --- |
| Frontal | Attention, thought, reasoning, behavior, movement, smell, and sexual urges |
| Parietal | Intellect, reasoning, touch, internal stimuli, language, reading, and visual functions |
| Temporal | Behavior, memory, hearing, visual functions, and emotions |
| Occipital | Vision |

separated by fissures. The functions of the cerebellum relate to balance and subconscious skeletal muscle movements, allowing the body to perform well-coordinated movements. The cerebellum is linked to the balance system of the inner ear to maintain equilibrium. A tumor in the cerebellum may result in symptoms relating to lack of balance and uncoordinated movement but, unlike the cerebral hemispheres, the symptoms affect the same side of the body as the damaged lobe.

The *diencephalon* is composed of the thalamus and hypothalamus, which interpret sensations such as touch, pressure, pain, and temperature. The hypothalamus monitors the body's internal environment, including blood temperature, hormone levels, and fluid levels. It also controls the autonomic nervous system and is the link between the nervous and endocrine systems, maintaining homeostasis.

The *brainstem* is composed of the midbrain, pons, and medulla oblongata. The midbrain connects the cerebral hemispheres. Posteriorly, the midbrain has four rounded eminences that are the reflex centers for sight and hearing. Below this lies the pons, which is composed mainly of nerve fibers passing between the cerebral hemispheres and also between the cerebral hemispheres and the spinal cord. Anatomically, the medulla oblongata is the inferior part of the brain and connects the brain to the spinal cord. In the medulla oblongata, nerve fibers from the cerebrum cross, which accounts for the fact that symptoms of disease can occur on the side of the body opposite that of the brain affected. This is known as the split-brain concept. The other functions of the medulla oblongata are related to consciousness and arousal as well as the vital reflex centers for respiratory, cardiac, and vasomotor functions.

For protection, the brain and spinal cord are covered by three membranes called *meninges* (Fig. 4.5). Cranial *dura mater* has two layers: an outer layer that adheres to the cranium (bone) and is known as the periosteal layer, and an inner layer known as the meningeal layer.

The cerebellum and cerebrum are separated by a fold of dura mater called the tentorium cerebelli (see Fig. 4.3). This tentorium is an anatomical division useful in distinguishing between the malignant pathologies of the CNS. Supratentorial tumors are confined to the cerebrum, and infratentorial tumors arise in the cerebellum or brainstem. The *pia mater* covers the brain, and the

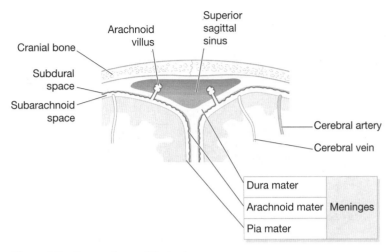

**Figure 4.5**   The meninges of the brain.

*arachnoid mater* between the dura mater and pia mater contains blood vessels. Further protection is afforded by cerebrospinal fluid (CSF), a clear colorless fluid secreted by a vascular fold of pia mater called the choroid plexus, which fills the subarachnoid space and bathes the spinal cord (Fig. 4.6). CSF also has a circulatory function, transporting nutrients from the blood to the brain and spinal cord and excreting waste products from the brain and spinal cord to the blood. The flow of CSF around the brain and spinal cord allows metastatic cells from tumors within the CNS to circulate throughout the system, which means that treatment may have to include the entire cerebrospinal axis.

The blood supply to the brain is vital for it to function. Oxygen and glucose, in particular, are vital to cell survival, and these pass quickly from the capillaries to the brain cells. Other substances in the blood do not enter as quickly, and some—for example, proteins and some drugs—do not enter at all because the capillaries of the brain are different in structure from those in the rest of the body. The cells are densely packed and have large numbers of glial cells surrounding them. This is known as the blood–brain barrier. The blood–brain barrier is useful in preventing harmful substances from entering the brain, but this also means that chemotherapy drugs are not always an effective method of treatment, as not all drugs will get through this 'barrier'.

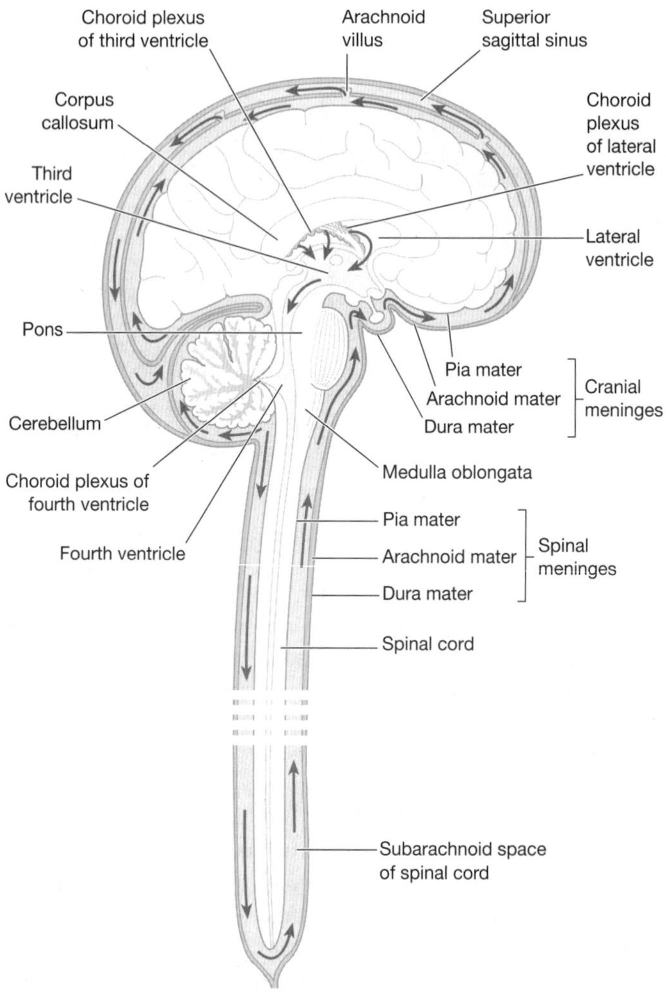

**Figure 4.6** The brain, spinal cord, and meninges, with flow of CSF indicated by arrows.

## The spinal cord

The spinal cord lies in the upper two thirds of the vertebral canal, extending from the upper border of the first cervical vertebra to the lower border of the first lumbar vertebra. The spinal cord is about 43 cm long in women and 45 cm long in men and is protected by the vertebral column. Nerves arise in pairs from a series of segments of the spinal cord which are named according to the vertebrae from which they arise. There are 31 pairs in total: 8 cervical, 12 thoracic, 5 lumbar, 5 sacral and 1 coccygeal. Since the spinal cord stops at the first lumbar vertebra, nerves that branch from the cord into lumbar and sacral levels run in the vertebral canal for some distance before they exit. This area is known as the cauda equina, where the nerves that supply the lower part of the body originate higher in the spinal cord, giving rise to symptoms at a distance from an area that is damaged or diseased. For example, the nerves controlling the muscles of the thigh originate at the second lumbar vertebra.

## ONCOLOGY

Primary CNS tumors are uncommon, accounting for 1–2% of all cancers worldwide each year. The overall male:female ratio is 1.5:1, with 90% of tumors arising in the brain and only 10% arising in the spinal cord. A bimodal pattern of incidence with age (with peaks under 10 years and at 55–80 years) occurs in CNS tumors. The majority of adults develop supratentorial tumors, while the majority of tumors in children are infratentorial. At least one third of all tumors are secondary or metastatic deposits from other primary sites, including breast and bronchus tumors.

The etiology of brain tumors is generally unknown, although causative factors may include ionizing radiation, occupational carcinogens, petrochemicals, agricultural work, and exposures in the rubber industry.

The primary histological types are not of neurons, but of supporting tissues and glands. Tumors arising from neurons are extremely rare. Eighty-five percent of primary tumors are gliomas arising from a malignant change in mature glial cells. These are named according to the glial cell type affected (see Table 4.1) and include astrocytomas, ependymomas, oligodendrogliomas, and medulloblastomas.

*Astrocytomas* are the most common histological type and arise from astrocytes, a type of supporting cell in the brain. They grow by direct extension into surrounding tissue. Classification is based on the histological features of the tumor and is reported on a four-grade scale used by the World Health Organization. These features are cellular pleomorphism (different cell shapes), mitotic activity (the

number of cells undergoing cell division), microvascular proliferation (increase in the number of blood vessels), and necrosis (cell
death). Grade I is the least malignant and has none of these features,
whereas grade IV—for example, glioblastoma multiforme—has
three or four of the features. Low grade astrocytomas are commonly found in the frontal, parietal, and temporal lobes of adults
and the brainstem and cerebellum of children. Astrocytomas can
occur supra- or infratentorially. A biopsy will not always give a
clear histological diagnosis of the whole tumor, as mixed varieties
are common. If the tumor is highly malignant, it may be impossible
to recognize the initial cell of origin. Initially, malignant tumors
invade the white matter and then the gray matter, though spread
throughout the CNS is rare.

*Ependymomas* account for 5% of all intracranial tumors and
occur mainly in childhood and early adulthood. They are derived
from the ciliated lining cells of the CNS cavities, which aid in the
circulation of CSF, and therefore commonly spread by seeding
throughout the CNS via the CSF. Over half arise from infratentorial sites, the most common site for childhood brain tumors.

*Oligodendrogliomas,* which are derived from oligodendrocytes,
typically arise supratentorially in the frontal, parietal, or temporal
lobes. Oligodendrogliomas are most common in adults and usually have a long, indolent history. The characteristic deposits of
calcium can be seen on a radiograph and aid in differential diagnosis. When spread via the CSF occurs, it is usually associated
with a rapidly growing and occasionally fatal tumor.

*Medulloblastomas* are derived from the fetal external layer of
the cerebellum that does not normally remain in the body after
birth. They are also known as primitive neuroectodermal tumors
(PNET) and account for 7–8% of intracranial tumors. They occur
predominantly in childhood, mainly in the cerebellum and therefore infratentorially. They metastasize via the CSF to the spinal
cord or other parts of the brain. Occasionally (fewer than 10% of
cases) there can be extraneural metastases.

Other tumors that can arise within the CNS include chordomas,
tumors of the pineal region, intracerebral lymphomas, and
tumors of the cranial nerves. Chordomas arise from the primitive
notochord, which in the embryo is tissue in a position where the
vertebral column will develop. This tissue normally disappears as
the fetus develops. Chordomas usually occur at the upper or lower

end of the spinal cord. Histologically, they look benign, but they invade local structures, and extensive bone destruction can occur. Tumors of the pineal region include malignant tumors such as dysgerminomas and pineoblastomas, both of which tend to spread via the CSF. Intracerebral lymphomas are very rare but have increased in incidence in recent years as one of the AIDS-related malignancies. As mentioned previously, tumors of nerve cells are rare because of their inability to divide; however, when they do occur, they tend to be benign. For example, acoustic neuromas arise from the VIIIth cranial nerve, which conveys impulses associated with hearing. Acoustic neuroma occurs in adults and is a benign slow-growing tumor causing unilateral deafness, vertigo, and tinnitus. Other cranial nerve tumors include ganglioneuroma and ganglioglioma. These tumors are dangerous because they create local pressure and related symptoms.

Brain tumors are classified on the basis of tumor cell type and histological grade. For some tumors, location and metastatic spread within the CSF are also used in classification. There is no tumor–node–metastasis (TNM) staging system for CNS tumors.

## Spread of intracranial tumors

Primary tumors of the CNS spread by local invasion. Metastatic spread outside the CNS is a rare occurrence mainly, it is thought, because of the lack of lymphatic drainage. Another reason may be that symptoms in this enclosed system tend to present early before spread outside has occurred. Metastatic spread outside the CNS is likely however via the CSF if ventriculoperitoneal shunting has been performed to relieve hydrocephalus. Seeding of cells via the CSF can result in multiple deposits on the surface of the brain and spinal cord. This is typical of medulloblastoma, ependymoma, and pineoblastoma, which means that treatment has to include the entire cerebrospinal axis.

On the other hand, metastatic spread to the CNS from other sites in the body, such as from tumors of the breast and bronchus, occurs commonly. These tumor cells appear to be able to cross the blood–brain barrier. However, this difference could be explained by the fact that primary brain tumors become symptomatic before cells cross the blood–brain barrier, rather than in terms of greater permeability to one malignant cell type than to another.

## Spinal tumors

Spinal tumors are classified by their site of origin within the meninges (Fig. 4.6) as extradural, intradural, or intramedullary. Extramedullary tumors tend to be metastatic disease; intradural tumors include meningiomas and neurofibromas; and intramedullary tumors include astrocytomas, ependymomas, and hemangioblastomas. Tumors often present with symptoms of spinal cord compression, which is seen when the lesion lies between the foramen magnum and the lower limit of the cord, or cauda equina compression when the lesion is below the limit of the spinal cord and affects only nerve roots. As mentioned earlier, spinal nerves emerge from the spinal cord higher than the area they supply; therefore symptoms of spinal cord compression can include lower limb paralysis.

## Clinical features

Clinical features can arise either from pressure caused by the tumor or from the location of the tumor within the CNS. As mentioned earlier, signs and symptoms will be related to the functions of different areas of the brain (see Table 4.3).

With the exception of tumors in the cerebellum, the symptoms and impairment appear on the opposite side of the body from

**Table 4.3**   Clinical features of tumors of the CNS

| Cause of clinical feature | Description of clinical feature |
| --- | --- |
| Increased intracranial pressure | Headache, vomiting, papilledema, drowsiness, mental deterioration, and personality changes |
| Cerebellar tumor | Loss of coordination of movement; headaches and vomiting |
| Frontal lobe tumor | Intellectual impairment and personality change; weakness and paralysis |
| Temporal lobe tumor | Epilepsy, speech disturbance, and visual field defects |
| Parietal lobe tumor | Sensory or visual inattention, difficulty with writing and simple mathematics |
| Occipital lobe tumor | Visual field defects, hallucinations, and seizures |
| Brainstem tumor | Cranial nerve defects, involvement of motor and sensory tracts |

the tumor location, because of the crossover of nerve fibers in the medulla oblongata.

## Investigations

Investigations for CNS tumors include contrast-enhanced computed tomography (CT) and magnetic resonance imaging (MRI) scans, stereotactic percutaneous needle biopsy or open biopsy and lumbar puncture for cerebral tumors, and myelogram and open biopsy for spinal tumors.

## Treatment

Management of CNS tumors depends on whether they are intracranial tumors (supratentorial or infratentorial) or spinal tumors and on the likelihood of spread throughout the system via the CSF. Surgery is recommended for most primary intracranial and spinal tumors if the lesion is accessible without causing neurological problems. Radiotherapy also has a major role in most tumor types and can increase disease-free survival. Surgery and radiotherapy can be used either alone or in combination. In cases where there is no evidence of seeding throughout the CNS, surgery will be followed by radiotherapy to the tumor bed or residual tumor only. Where there is evidence of, or the likelihood of, seeding via the CSF, such as in medulloblastoma and ependymoma, the entire CNS will require radiotherapy. This entails treating the brain and spinal cord. This is complex radiotherapy treatment requiring careful shielding of organs within the head and neck region that do not require treatment, for example the eyes and mouth. For patients with metastatic disease to the brain, the whole brain will be treated with radiotherapy to relieve symptoms. If brain irradiation is planned, the patient will have an individual perspex mask made, which will be worn during treatment to enable the head to remain still throughout the procedure.

Chemotherapy is not commonly used, because drugs (with the exception of some lipid-soluble agents) are unable to cross the blood–brain barrier. Drugs can be injected into the CSF via a lumbar puncture (intrathecally), but care must be taken not to spread the disease by using this method. Supportive therapy can be given in the form of steroids to relieve the symptoms of increased intracranial pressure.

## Prognosis

The prognosis of tumors of the CNS depends on their grade, histological type, and extent. Grade I astrocytomas have a 5-year survival of 50–85%, but this drops to less than 10% for grade IV. Similar trends can be seen in other histological types. Well differentiated oligodendrogliomas have a 5-year survival of 75%, dropping to less than 45% if anaplastic; for medulloblastomas, 5-year survival is in the range 25–70%.

## SELF-ASSESSMENT QUESTIONS

Answer true or false to the following. Answers are on page 243.

1. The central nervous system comprises the brain and spinal cord.
2. Neurons can renew themselves indefinitely.
3. Glial cells are the supporting cells of the CNS.
4. The CNS maintains homeostasis in the body.
5. Myelin gives the gray appearance to neural matter.
6. The cerebellum is the largest component of the brain.
7. The cerebral hemispheres are divided into five lobes.
8. The right cerebral hemisphere is important for left hand control.
9. The occipital lobe is concerned with balance.
10. The spinal cord runs throughout the length of the vertebral column.
11. Primary tumors of the CNS are uncommon.
12. Tumors arising from neurons are common.
13. Astrocytoma is the most common histology of primary CNS tumors.
14. Ependymomas are derived from ciliated lining cells of CNS cavities.
15. Infratentorial tumors occur mostly in adults.
16. Spread outside the CNS from a brain primary is common.
17. Signs and symptoms depend on the site of the tumor.
18. Metastatic disease to the brain is common.
19. Chemotherapy is the treatment of choice.
20. Prognosis is dependent on the grade of the tumor.

# 5

# The endocrine system

Two regulatory systems, the nervous system and the endocrine system, work together to maintain equilibrium (homeostasis) of bodily functions. The endocrine system is made up of a series of glands (Fig. 5.1) that secrete hormones directly into the bloodstream to be dispersed throughout the body. This makes them different from exocrine glands that secrete their products into ducts, which in turn transfer them to a body cavity. Hormones are designed to target many different areas of the body. Generally, hormones affect the metabolic rate of cells—that is, how quickly or slowly they break down or re-form the chemicals necessary for cellular survival.

The endocrine glands to be covered in this chapter include the pituitary gland, thyroid gland, and the adrenal glands. Other organs of the body, such as the small intestine, pancreas, testes, and ovary, also contain endocrine tissue. The endocrine functions of these organs are covered in other chapters.

## THE PITUITARY GLAND (HYPOPHYSIS)

The pituitary gland lies centrally within the sella turcica of the skull in a protected position (Fig. 5.2). The deepest part of the sella turcica is often referred to as the pituitary fossa since the pituitary gland sits in it. The gland is connected to the base of the brain via a stalk called the infundibulum. Immediately superior to the pituitary gland lies the optic chiasma, where the optic nerves cross. This area can be related to common presenting symptoms for pituitary tumors (see below). The pituitary is composed of an anterior

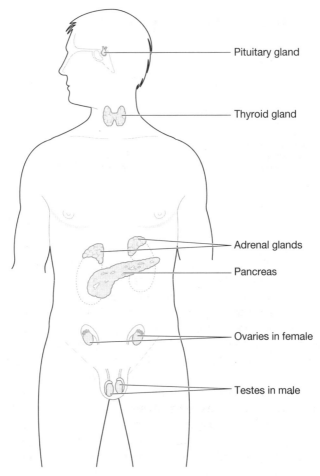

Pituitary gland

Thyroid gland

Adrenal glands

Pancreas

Ovaries in female

Testes in male

**Figure 5.1**   The endocrine system.

lobe, which is glandular tissue and is sometimes referred to as the adenohypophysis, and a posterior lobe, which is nervous tissue and is referred to as the neurohypophysis.

Microscopically, the anterior pituitary is made up of three types of cells, named according to their affinity for certain staining techniques or lack thereof. Chromophobe cells do not stain; acidophil cells, sometimes referred to as eosinophils, stain red; and basophil cells stain blue. Table 5.1 lists the hormones which are produced by these cells, and their principal target organs.

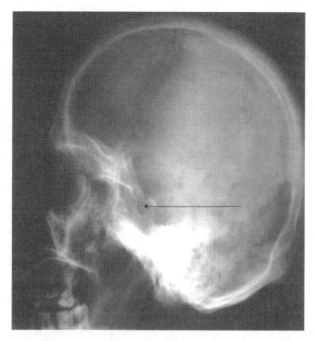

**Figure 5.2**    Lateral skull radiograph demonstrating the position of the pituitary gland in the sella turcica.

**Table 5.1**    Anterior pituitary hormones and their target organs

| Type of cell producing hormone | Hormone | Target organ |
| --- | --- | --- |
| Acidophil (eosinophil) | Growth hormone | Bone, muscle |
| | Prolactin | Breast |
| Basophil | Thyroid-stimulating hormone | Thyroid gland |
| | Follicle-stimulating hormone | Ovaries, testes |
| | Luteinizing hormone | Ovaries, testes |
| | Melanocyte-stimulating hormone | Skin |
| | Adrenocorticotropic hormone | Adrenal cortex |
| Chromophobe | None | None |

The posterior pituitary is a storage area for hormones produced in the hypothalamus. The cells which store the hormones are called pituicytes. Two hormones are released from the posterior pituitary gland: antidiuretic hormone and oxytocin.

## Oncology

Virtually all tumors of the pituitary gland arise from the anterior lobe and are invariably benign and curable. Pituitary adenomas present a danger to the individual mainly because of the proximity to vital structures. Any of the tumors may enlarge the sella turcica, causing pressure symptoms. Pressure on the optic chiasma causes visual defects, and pressure on the brain may even cause death. Clinical syndromes may also be present with hormonally active tumors. Eosinophilic tumors often secrete growth hormone, resulting in gigantism in younger patients and acromegaly in others. Basophilic tumors secrete prolactin and adrenocorticotropic hormone, resulting in Cushing's syndrome.

### Staging

There is no TNM staging scheme for pituitary cancers.

### Treatment

Magnetic resonance imaging now plays an important role in localizing these tumors, but plain film radiography and computed tomography still have a role. The mainstay of treatment is trans-sphenoidal surgery, particularly for those tumors confined to the sella turcica. Any extension beyond the sella turcica may be an indication for external beam radiotherapy. Non-functioning chromophobe adenomas tend to extend beyond the confines of the sella turcica, and extra radiation therapy is therefore indicated. Bromocriptine has been successful as a medical treatment for prolactin-secreting tumors, and somatostatin analogs can be used for those tumors secreting growth hormone.

## THE THYROID GLAND

The thyroid gland is located just below the larynx (Fig. 5.3). The thyroid consists of a right and left lobe either side of the trachea, joined by a mass of tissue on the anterior aspect of the trachea called the isthmus. Histologically, the thyroid is composed of spherical sacs called thyroid follicles, and the walls of each follicle consist of two types of cells: follicular and parafollicular (C) cells. The follicular cells produce two hormones, thyroxine ($T_4$) and triiodothyronine ($T_3$). These

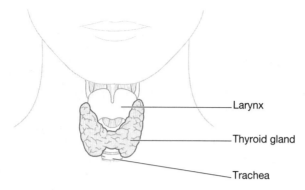

Larynx

Thyroid gland

Trachea

**Figure 5.3**    The thyroid gland.

hormones help regulate metabolism and the process of growth and tissue differentiation. The thyroid has a very rich blood supply and is relatively close to the carotid artery. Lymphatic drainage is primarily to the cervical lymph nodes and the pre- and paratracheal nodes, and lymphatic drainage continues inferiorly to the mediastinum. Running down the side of the thyroid gland is the recurrent laryngeal nerve.

## Oncology

Thyroid cancer is rare, but it is the most common form of endocrine tumor. It is a disease that is slightly more common in women, and can affect a wide range of ages (commonly between 25 and 65 years). Malignant tumors of the thyroid usually have one of four main histologies: papillary carcinoma, follicular carcinoma, medullary carcinoma, or anaplastic carcinoma. Lymphomas and sarcomas are uncommon.

*Papillary carcinoma* is the most common form of thyroid cancer, most cases of which will present as multifocal disease throughout the thyroid gland. Spread to brain and bone does occur at a late stage but more commonly spread is via the lymphatic system to the cervical lymph node chain.

*Follicular carcinoma*, along with papillary carcinoma, tends to be well differentiated, and about half of the tumors display the ability to utilize iodine to form thyroid hormone, although this occurs more commonly in follicular than in papillary tumors. Ingestion of radio-iodine plays an important role in the treatment of patients with this condition. Normally, well differentiated follicular tumors are well circumscribed. It is important at diagnosis to distinguish these from their benign counterpart, follicular adenoma. Spread to lymph nodes is fairly common, but this does not reduce survival. Follicular tumors readily spread via the blood to lungs and bone.

*Medullary carcinoma* arises from the parafollicular cells of the thyroid and constitutes 5–10% of all thyroid cancers. These cancers can be sporadic in nature, and tend to be confined to one lobe of the thyroid. Medullary carcinoma may be familial in nature. These cancers are almost always bilateral at presentation and may be associated with multiple endocrine neoplasia (MEN) syndrome, in which other endocrine organs are affected. If familial medullary carcinoma is suspected, other members of the family should also be screened for disease. Familial medullary tumors may secrete calcitonin, which can be used as a tumor marker to monitor the efficacy of treatment. Spread to the cervical and mediastinal lymph nodes is common.

An *anaplastic tumor* is a highly aggressive, undifferentiated tumor. Spread via blood is early, but invasion of local tissues causes the main problems with this tumor. The trachea can be breached, causing stridor, or the esophagus, causing dysphagia. Invasion of the recurrent laryngeal nerve may cause pain, and a breach of the carotid artery can cause death. Anaplastic tumors may be subclassified into small cell and large cell. If small cell is suspected, this must be distinguished from lymphoma of the thyroid gland.

### Staging

It is important to know the histology of the disease when staging thyroid carcinoma. Box 5.1 and Table 5.2 give TNM definitions and stage groups.

### Treatment

Papillary and follicular tumors are best treated with surgery. Treatment may be lobectomy or total thyroidectomy and is largely dependent on the localized extent of the tumor and the age of the patient. Because of the likely functioning nature of the disease, radio-iodine may be administered to ablate any remaining thyroid tissue, in order to reduce the chance of recurrence. Lifelong supportive therapy in the form of replacement thyroid hormone is necessary.

---

**Box 5.1**   Thyroid carcinoma—TNM definitions

**Primary tumor (T)**
Note: All categories may be subdivided into (a) solitary tumor or (b) multifocal tumor (the largest determines the classification)
- TX: Primary tumor cannot be assessed
- T0: No evidence of primary tumor
- T1: Tumor 2 cm or less in greatest dimension limited to the thyroid
- T2: Tumor more than 2 cm but not more than 4 cm in greatest dimension limited to the thyroid
- T3: Tumor more than 4 cm in greatest dimension limited to the thyroid
- T4a: Tumor of any size extending beyond the thyroid capsule to invade subcutaneous soft tissues, larynx, trachea, esophagus, or recurrent laryngeal nerve
- T4b: Tumor invades prevertebral fascia or encases carotid artery or mediastinal vessels

All anaplastic carcinomas are considered T4 tumors:

- T4a: Intrathyroid anaplastic carcinoma—surgically resectable
- T4b: Intrathyroid anaplastic carcinoma—surgically unresectable

**Regional lymph node involvement (N)**
- NX: Regional lymph nodes cannot be assessed
- N0: No regional lymph node metastasis
- N1: Regional lymph node metastasis
  —N1a: Metastasis to level VI (pretracheal, paratracheal, and prelaryngeal/Delphian) lymph nodes
  —N1b: Metastasis in unilateral, bilateral, or contralateral cervical or superior mediastinal lymph nodes

**Distant metastasis (M)**
- MX: Distant metastasis cannot be assessed
- M0: No distant metastasis
- M1: Distant metastasis

---

Family members suspected of having medullary carcinoma should be screened for raised calcitonin level and the presence of the *RET* proto-oncogene as an important strategy for improved survival. Many of the patients with medullary carcinoma have lymph node spread to cervical and mediastinal regions. Total thyroidectomy is advocated for medullary carcinoma, along with en bloc neck dissection. These tumors are rarely functional; radioiodine has little efficacy.

Anaplastic tumors are locally very destructive. Surgery is advocated if the tumor remains localized, but this is rare. The most common treatment involves external beam radiotherapy.

Patients with well differentiated tumors (normally papillary and follicular) have a favorable prognosis, with many surviving 10 years. Patients with anaplastic tumors have a poor survival rate.

**Table 5.2** Thyroid carcinoma—stage groups

| Stage | Primary tumor | Regional node involvement | Distant metastasis |
|---|---|---|---|
| *Papillary or follicular carcinoma, under 45 years* | | | |
| I | Any T | Any N | M0 |
| II | Any T | Any N | M1 |
| *Papillary or follicular carcinoma, over 45 years* | | | |
| I | T1 | N0 | M0 |
| II | T2 | N0 | M0 |
| III | T3 | N0 | M0 |
| | T1 | N1a | M0 |
| | T2 | N1a | M0 |
| | T3 | N1a | M0 |
| IVA | T4a | N0 | M0 |
| | T4a | N1a | M0 |
| | T1 | N1b | M0 |
| | T2 | N1b | M0 |
| | T3 | N1b | M0 |
| | T4a | N1b | M0 |
| IVB | T4b | Any N | M0 |
| IVC | Any T | Any N | M1 |
| *Medullary carcinoma* | | | |
| I | T1 | N0 | M0 |
| II | T2 | N0 | M0 |
| III | T3 | N0 | M0 |
| | T1 | N1a | M0 |
| | T2 | N1a | M0 |
| | T3 | N1a | M0 |
| IVA | T4a | N0 | M0 |
| | T4a | N1a | M0 |
| | T1 | N1b | M0 |
| | T2 | N1b | M0 |
| | T3 | N1b | M0 |
| | T4a | N1b | M0 |
| IVB | T4b | Any N | M0 |
| IVC | Any T | Any N | M1 |
| *Anaplastic carcinoma—all anaplastic carcinomas are considered to be stage IV* | | | |
| IVA | T4a | Any N | M0 |
| IVB | T4b | Any N | M0 |
| IVC | Any T | Any N | M1 |

With medullary carcinoma, patients who have been diagnosed through screening have a better chance of survival.

# ADRENAL GLANDS

The adrenal glands are located immediately superior to the kidneys (Fig. 5.4). They are divided structurally and functionally into

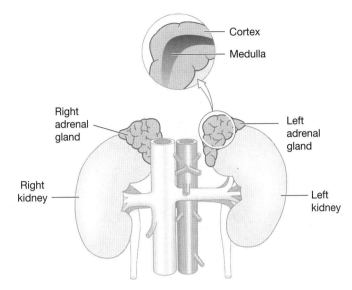

**Figure 5.4**   The adrenal glands.

two parts: an outer section called the cortex and an inner one called the medulla.

The adrenal cortex secretes mainly glucocorticoid hormones such as hydrocortisone and cortisone. It also secretes aldosterone and small amounts of sex hormones. Over-secretion of these hormones is common in approximately 60% of adrenal cortex tumors, and patients may present with a variety of syndromes such as Cushing's syndrome, adrenogenital syndrome, virilization, hyperaldosteronism, and feminization. Adrenal cortex carcinoma is rare, and treatment consists mainly of surgery. Postoperative radiotherapy has shown some benefit, as has the chemotherapy drug mitotane (Lysodren) for later stage disease.

The adrenal medulla secretes epinephrine (adrenaline) and norepinephrine (noradrenaline), which are hormones that act in the 'fight or flight' response of the body. *Pheochromocytoma* is the tumor most often identified in the adrenal medulla. Pheochromocytoma is often associated with increased secretion of the adrenal medulla hormones, and this is often used to diagnose the disease. Unfortunately, pheochromocytoma may be benign or malignant, and histologically it is difficult to tell them apart. Nevertheless, the treatment of choice is surgical removal, with associated regional lymph nodes if spread had been detected. Bilateral tumors affect a small percentage of patients, and these are usually associated with MEN, as outlined earlier. Identification of MEN calls for regular family screening for this disease.

## Staging

There is no TNM staging scheme for adrenal gland carcinoma.

## Prognosis

Patients diagnosed with adrenal gland tumors early have a good chance of survival. If spread is detected to local lymph nodes or further, the prognosis is worsened.

# SELF-ASSESSMENT QUESTIONS

Answer true or false to the following. Answers are on page 244.

1. Endocrine glands secrete mucus.
2. The pituitary is situated below the optic chiasma.
3. The pituitary gland is situated in a recess of the sphenoid bone of the skull.
4. The pituitary gland is also referred to as the hypophysis.
5. Virtually all tumors of the pituitary gland are malignant.
6. Acidophilic adenoma is a hormone-secreting tumor.
7. Benign pituitary tumor can be life-threatening.
8. The thyroid gland lies posterior to the larynx.
9. Lymphatic drainage of the thyroid is primarily to the cervical lymph node chain.
10. The thyroid gland uses thyroxine to produce its hormones.
11. Papillary carcinoma is the most common form of thyroid tumor.
12. Anaplastic tumors of the thyroid are usually very slow-growing.
13. Radioactive iodine is often used in the treatment of all thyroid tumors.
14. Medullary carcinoma of the thyroid has familial tendencies.
15. A T2 tumor of the thyroid is defined as being 2–4 cm in size.
16. Papillary and follicular tumors of the thyroid are usually well differentiated.
17. The adrenal glands are located inferior to the kidneys.
18. The adrenal glands are divided into an outer cortex and an inner medulla.
19. Pheochromocytoma is a tumor most commonly associated with the adrenal cortex.
20. Pheochromocytoma may be benign or malignant.

# The respiratory system

This chapter deals with the pharynx, larynx, bronchi, and lungs.

## THE PHARYNX

Anatomically the pharynx (Fig. 6.1) is divided into three sections. The *nasopharynx* lies posterior to the nasal cavity and extends from the base of the skull inferiorly to the level of the soft palate. It is continuous with the *oropharynx*, which lies posterior to the mouth and extends inferiorly to the level of the hyoid bone. Inferior to this is the *laryngopharynx* (hypopharynx) which extends from the level of the hyoid bone to its termination in the esophagus, posterior to the larynx.

Several openings can be found in the pharynx:

- right and left auditory tubes opening into the nasopharynx
- two posterior nares from the nasal cavity into the nasopharynx
- the opening of the mouth (fauces) into the oropharynx
- the opening of the larynx and esophagus from the laryngopharynx.

Each of these openings plays a part in the potential spread of tumors within this region, and the signs and symptoms with which patients present can often be traced back to involvement of these structures. Similarly there is a deep depression posterior to the openings of the auditory tubes called the fossa of Rosenmüller, and this is a common site of presentation of nasopharyngeal tumors.

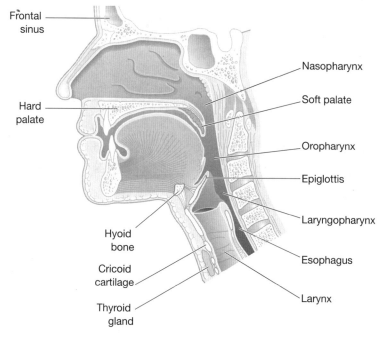

Frontal sinus

Hard palate

Hyoid bone

Cricoid cartilage

Thyroid gland

Nasopharynx

Soft palate

Oropharynx

Epiglottis

Laryngopharynx

Esophagus

Larynx

**Figure 6.1** Anatomy of the pharynx.

Functionally, the pharynx plays a role in both the respiratory and digestive systems. It also plays an important part in the creation of sounds.

An important source of aggregated lymphatic tissue, collectively known as the tonsils, is located in this region. Three pairs of tonsils are sometimes referred to as Waldeyer's ring, and protect the passageway from harmful microorganisms. The pharyngeal tonsils are located on the posterior wall of the nasopharynx opposite the posterior nares. The palatine tonsils in the oropharynx are located behind and below the pillars of fauces, and the lingual tonsils are located at the base of the tongue. The epithelial lining of the pharynx changes slightly from a pseudostratified ciliated columnar form in the nasopharynx to a stratified squamous form in the laryngopharynx.

The pharynx has a rich lymphatic drainage, and as a result early lymphatic involvement is common. Of importance is the node of Rouviere which is found in the lateral aspect of the retropharyngeal wall, and is a point of early involvement particularly for nasopharyngeal tumors. Other directions of lymphatic spread can be to the jugulodigastric nodes, jugulo-omohyoid, deep cervical chain, and the posterior triangle.

# Oncology

## Nasopharyngeal carcinoma

Nasopharyngeal carcinoma is rare in most parts of the world, but is relatively common in parts of southeast Asia. The highest incidence worldwide occurs in people of Chinese origin. Some forms of the cancer are also associated with the Epstein–Barr virus (EBV), and in rare cases nasopharyngeal carcinoma has a tendency to run in families. Possible causes include exposure to nitrosamines, polycyclic hydrocarbons, chronic nasal infection, poor hygiene, and poor ventilation of the nasopharynx. Unlike other head and neck cancers, alcohol and smoking do not tend to be associated with nasopharyngeal carcinoma. Generally, more males than females are affected.

The main presenting pathology is squamous cell carcinoma (SCC), although this cell type is often subdivided into well and poorly differentiated tumors, with anaplastic tumors making up a third variety. Because there is also an abundance of lymphatic tissue in this region, lymphomas, usually of the non-Hodgkin variety, are also quite common.

Patients may present with a variety of signs and symptoms. Occlusion of the eustachian tube may lead to hearing difficulties, cranial nerve dysfunction (usually II–VI or IX–XII), enlarged cervical lymph nodes (which may be bilateral because of the cross-lymphatic drainage of this area), sore throat, epistaxis, or blocked nose.

**Staging**   Box 6.1 and Table 6.1 give the TNM definitions and stage groups for nasopharyngeal carcinoma.

**Treatment**   Radiotherapy remains the treatment of choice for tumors in the nasopharyngeal region, whether they be of squamous epithelial type or lymphomas. Generally, SCCs will receive higher doses of radiation than lymphomas. Radiotherapy for SCCs tends to involve the primary site along with potential routes of spread. The upper deep cervical lymph node chain should be included in the field along with the nodes of the posterior triangle and lateral pharyngeal area. Both sides of the head and neck should be treated because of the likelihood of cross-lymphatic spread.

---

**Box 6.1** Nasopharyngeal carcinoma—TNM definitions

**Primary tumor (T)**
- TX: Primary tumor cannot be assessed
- T0: No evidence of primary tumor
- Tis: Carcinoma in situ
- T1: Tumor confined to the nasopharynx
- T2: Tumor extends to soft tissues of oropharynx and/or nasal cavity
  —T2a: without parapharyngeal extension[a]
  —T2b: with parapharyngeal extension[a]
- T3: Tumor invades bony structures and/or paranasal sinuses
- T4: Tumor with intracranial extension and/or involvement of cranial nerves, infratemporal fossa, hypopharynx, orbit, or masticator space

**Regional lymph node involvement (N)**
- NX: Regional lymph nodes cannot be assessed
- N0: No regional lymph node metastasis
- N1: Unilateral metastasis in lymph node(s), 6 cm or less in greatest dimension, above the supraclavicular fossa[b]
- N2: Bilateral metastasis in lymph node(s), 6 cm or less in greatest dimension, above the supraclavicular fossa[b]
- N3: Metastasis in lymph node(s)[b] >6 cm and/or to supraclavicular fossa:[c]
  —N3a: >6 cm
  —N3b: extension to the supraclavicular fossa[c]

**Distant metastasis (M)**
- MX: Distant metastasis cannot be assessed
- M0: No distant metastasis
- M1: Distant metastasis

---

[a] Parapharyngeal extension denotes posterolateral infiltration of tumor beyond the pharyngobasilar fascia.
[b] Midline nodes are considered ipsilateral nodes.
[c] Supraclavicular zone or fossa is relevant to the staging of nasopharyngeal carcinoma and is the triangular region originally described by Ho. It is defined by three points: (1) the superior margin of the sternal end of the clavicle, (2) the superior margin of the lateral end of the clavicle, (3) the point where the neck meets the shoulder. Note that this would include caudal portions of levels IV and V. All cases with lymph nodes (whole or part) in the fossa are considered N3b.

---

Doses of around 65 Gy in 32 fractions over 6–7 weeks can be given. Normally the cervical lymph nodes are shielded from the photon field after approximately 40 Gy and given an extra radiation dose using electrons. Lymphomas are more radiosensitive, and therefore lower doses of radiation are required. Generally, wide field regional radiotherapy is indicated, to include all of Waldeyer's ring and associated lymphatic drainage. Normal doses are in the region of 35–40 Gy in 20 fractions over 4 weeks.

**Table 6.1**  Nasopharyngeal carcinoma—stage groups

| Stage | Primary tumor | Regional node involvement | Distant metastasis |
|-------|---------------|---------------------------|--------------------|
| 0 | Tis | N0 | M0 |
| I | T1 | N0 | M0 |
| IIA | T2a | N0 | M0 |
| IIB | T1 | N1 | M0 |
| | T2 | N1 | M0 |
| | T2a | N1 | M0 |
| | T2b | N0 | M0 |
| | T2b | N1 | M0 |
| III | T1 | N2 | M0 |
| | T2a | N2 | M0 |
| | T2b | N2 | M0 |
| | T3 | N0 | M0 |
| | T3 | N1 | M0 |
| | T3 | N2 | M0 |
| IVA | T4 | N0 | M0 |
| | T4 | N1 | M0 |
| | T4 | N2 | M0 |
| IVB | Any T | N3 | M0 |
| IVC | Any T | Any N | M1 |

Sometimes brachytherapy is used to boost the dose to the primary site. The relatively inaccessible nature of the nasopharynx makes this a difficult procedure, and treatment of this type should only be attempted in specialized centers. Any surgical procedures are normally limited to biopsy.

**Prognosis**  Patients with early stage disease survive longer. Five-year survival rates in China range between 60% and 85% for stages I and II, but fall to around 30% for stages III and IV.

### Oropharyngeal carcinoma

Oropharyngeal carcinoma is also a rare disease in the UK. It is predominantly a disease of the elderly (median age is about 65 years). It is far more common in males than females, which may be related to habitual smoking and high alcohol intake. The use of mouthwash with high alcohol intake has also been implicated in an increase in oropharyngeal tumors. Squamous cell carcinoma is the predominant pathology. However, because of the abundance of lymphoid tissue present, non-Hodgkin lymphomas are also quite common.

---

**Box 6.2** Oropharyngeal carcinoma—TNM definitions

**Primary tumor (T)**
- TX: Primary tumor cannot be assessed
- T0: No evidence of primary tumor
- Tis: Carcinoma in situ
- T1: Tumor 2 cm or less in greatest dimension
- T2: Tumor more than 2 cm but not more than 4 cm in greatest dimension
- T3: Tumor more than 4 cm in greatest dimension
- T4: Tumor invades adjacent structures
  —T4a: Tumor invades the larynx, deep/extrinsic muscle of tongue, medial pterygoid, hard palate, or mandible
  —T4b: Tumor invades lateral pterygoid muscle, pterygoid plates, lateral nasopharynx, or skull base, or encases carotid artery

**Regional lymph node involvement (N)**
- NX: Regional lymph nodes cannot be assessed
- N0: No regional lymph node metastasis
- N1: Metastasis in a single ipsilateral lymph node, 3 cm or less in greatest dimension
- N2: Metastasis in a single ipsilateral lymph node, more than 3 cm but not more than 6 cm in greatest dimension, or in multiple ipsilateral lymph nodes, none more than 6 cm in greatest dimension, or in bilateral or contralateral lymph nodes, none more than 6 cm in greatest dimension
  —N2a: Metastasis in a single ipsilateral lymph node, more than 3 cm but not more than 6 cm in greatest dimension
  —N2b: Metastasis in multiple ipsilateral lymph nodes, none more than 6 cm in greatest dimension
  —N2c: Metastasis in bilateral or contralateral lymph nodes, none more than 6 cm in greatest dimension
- N3: Metastasis in a lymph node more than 6 cm in greatest dimension

**Distant metastasis (M)**
- MX: Distant metastasis cannot be assessed
- M0: No distant metastasis
- M1: Distant metastasis

---

Patients may present with a variety of symptoms, mainly associated with the tumor site of presentation and the local spread of the tumor. Base of tongue tumors may produce fixation of the tongue, resulting in slurring of speech. Referred pain to the ears may occur if spread superior to the eustachian tubes is present. Tonsillar tumors tend to present with no or mild pain and dysphagia as the tumor begins to occlude the passageway. Early lymph spread is common, with many patients presenting with node enlargement in the neck, some of which may be bilateral.

**Staging** TNM definitions and stage groups for oropharyngeal carcinoma are given in Box 6.2 and Table 6.2.

**Table 6.2** Oropharyngeal and hypopharyngeal (laryngopharyngeal) carcinoma—stage groups

| Stage | Primary tumor | Regional node involvement | Distant metastasis |
|---|---|---|---|
| 0 | Tis | N0 | M0 |
| I | T1 | N0 | M0 |
| II | T2 | N0 | M0 |
| III | T3 | N0 | M0 |
| | T1 | N1 | M0 |
| | T2 | N1 | M0 |
| | T3 | N1 | M0 |
| IVA | T4a | N0 | M0 |
| | T4a | N1 | M0 |
| | T1 | N2 | M0 |
| | T2 | N2 | M0 |
| | T3 | N2 | M0 |
| | T4a | N2 | M0 |
| IVB | T4b | Any N | M0 |
| | Any T | N3 | M0 |
| IVC | Any T | Any N | M1 |

**Treatment**   Neither external beam radiotherapy nor surgery has any predominant influence over survival. For early stage tumors surgery may be the preferred modality where the functional deficit will be minimal, such as the tonsillar pillar. If functional deficit is a cause of concern then external beam radiotherapy can be used. For later stages a combination of surgery and radiation is used. Chemoradiotherapy has been attempted but the results are inconclusive.

Lymphomas are more radiosensitive, and therefore lower doses of radiation are required. Generally, wide field regional radiotherapy is indicated, to include all of Waldeyer's ring and associated lymphatic drainage. Normal doses are in the region of 35–40 Gy in 20 fractions over 4 weeks.

**Prognosis**   Crude 5-year survival figures indicate that around 40% of all patients will survive.

## Laryngopharyngeal carcinoma

The laryngopharynx, or hypopharynx, extends from the plane of the hyoid bone distally to the plane of the lower border of the cricoid cartilage. It does not include the larynx. The hypopharynx has three parts: the pyriform fossa, the postcricoid area, and the posterior pharyngeal wall. The pyriform fossa is the most frequently involved site in the laryngopharynx. Postcricoid and posterior laryngopharyngeal wall carcinomas account for only one-third of laryngopharyngeal cancers.

When involved by cancer this anatomical region does not generate symptoms until late in the course of the disease. In addition to having a high incidence of early metastases, tumors of the laryngopharynx have survival rates that are perhaps the lowest of all sites in the head and neck. The predominant cell type is SCC. Often presentation is associated with a history of excess use of tobacco or alcohol. The Plummer–Vinson syndrome is frequently associated with carcinoma of the laryngopharynx, oral cavity, or esophagus in women. This syndrome is characterized by glossitis (inflammation of the tongue), iron deficiency anemia, and a congenital web of tissue which protrudes into the upper esophagus.

The lymphatic drainage from the pharynx is into the jugulodigastric, jugulo-omohyoid, upper and middle deep cervical, and retropharyngeal nodes. Cervical node metastasis is frequent, occurring in 70% of pyriform fossa lesions, 40% of postcricoid carcinomas, and 50% of posterior hypopharyngeal wall lesions.

**Staging** TNM definitions for laryngopharyngeal carcinoma are given in Box 6.3 and Table 6.2.

**Treatment** Because of the nature of this disease and its lack of symptoms until late in its course, it is unusual to have patients with early stage disease. As a consequence, the tumor tends to invade locally and early via the lymphatic system. Surgery is the mainstay of treatment for these patients, with total laryngopharyngectomy and neck dissection being the norm. For later stage disease, postoperative radiotherapy may be used. Neoadjuvant chemotherapy is sometimes used to shrink the tumor prior to administering other forms of treatment.

## THE LARYNX

The larynx or voice box (Fig. 6.2) lies below the hyoid bone, anterior to the esophagus and continuous with the trachea. It is supported by cartilages and contains the vocal fold (vocal cords). The function of the larynx is to produce sound that varies in pitch. This is achieved by varying the tension of the ligaments within the vocal fold. The width of the slit between the vocal folds can

---

**Box 6.3**    Hypopharyngeal (laryngopharyngeal) carcinoma—TNM definitions

**Primary tumor (T)**
- TX: Primary tumor cannot be assessed
- T0: No evidence of primary tumor
- Tis: Carcinoma in situ
- T1: Tumor limited to one subsite[a] of the hypopharynx and 2 cm or less in greatest dimension
- T2: Tumor involves more than one subsite[a] of the hypopharynx or an adjacent site, or measures more than 2 cm but not more than 4 cm in greatest diameter without fixation of hemilarynx
- T3: Tumor measures more than 4 cm in greatest dimension or with fixation of hemilarynx
- T4: Tumor invades adjacent structures
  —T4a: Tumor invades thyroid/cricoid cartilage, hyoid bone, thyroid gland, esophagus, or central compartment soft tissue[b]
  —T4b: Tumor invades prevertebral fascia, encases carotid artery, or involves mediastinal structures

**Regional lymph node involvement (N)**
- NX: Regional lymph nodes cannot be assessed
- N0: No regional lymph node metastasis
- N1: Metastasis in a single ipsilateral lymph node, 3 cm or less in greatest dimension
- N2: Metastasis in a single ipsilateral lymph node, more than 3 cm but not more than 6 cm in greatest dimension, or in multiple ipsilateral lymph nodes, none more than 6 cm in greatest dimension, or in bilateral or contralateral lymph nodes, none more than 6 cm in greatest dimension
  —N2a: Metastasis in a single ipsilateral lymph node, more than 3 cm but not more than 6 cm in greatest dimension
  —N2b: Metastasis in multiple ipsilateral lymph nodes, none more than 6 cm in greatest dimension
  —N2c: Metastasis in bilateral or contralateral lymph nodes, none more than 6 cm in greatest dimension
- N3: Metastasis in a lymph node more than 6 cm in greatest dimension

**Distant metastasis (M)**
- MX: Distant metastasis cannot be assessed
- M0: No distant metastasis
- M1: Distant metastasis

---

[a]Subsites of the hypopharynx are as follows:
- *pharyngo-esophageal junction* (postcricoid area), extending from the level of the arytenoid cartilages and connecting folds to the inferior border of the cricoid cartilage;
- *pyriform sinus*, extending from the pharyngo-epiglottic fold to the upper end of the esophagus, bounded laterally by the thyroid cartilage and medially by the surface of the aryepiglottic fold and the arytenoid and cricoid cartilages;
- *posterior pharyngeal wall*, extending from the level of the floor of the vallecula to the level of the crico-arytenoid joints.

[b]Central compartment soft tissue includes prelaryngeal strap muscles and subcutaneous fat.

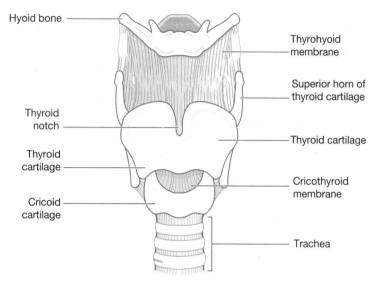

**Figure 6.2** Anatomy of the larynx.

also be varied by movement of the arytenoid cartilages brought about by the vocal muscles. Anatomically, the larynx is divided into three regions. The supraglottic region (supraglottis) includes the epiglottis, false vocal cords, ventricles, aryepiglottic folds, and arytenoids. The glottic region (glottis) includes the true vocal cords and the anterior and posterior commissures. The subglottic region (subglottis) begins about 1 cm below the true vocal cords and extends to the lower border of the cricoid cartilage.

Knowledge of the lymphatic drainage of the larynx is important in understanding the presentation and associated management of malignant disease arising in this area. The true vocal cords have sparse lymphatic drainage, which explains why true vocal cord tumors rarely present with cervical lymph node enlargement. By contrast, the supraglottic and subglottic regions have a rich lymphatic network. The supraglottic region drains principally to the upper deep cervical lymph node chain, and a great proportion of patients with malignant disease will present with enlarged nodes. The subglottic region drains to the paratracheal and lower cervical nodes. Mediastinal lymph node involvement is considered distant metastasis.

# Oncology

Cancer of the larynx is one of the most common head and neck cancers in Europe. Because changes in voice and a sore throat tend to be common presenting symptoms, patients are likely to seek medical advice early. As a consequence, most of the tumors tend to be of an early stage at presentation. Approximately three-quarters of tumors will occur in the glottic region (vocal folds) of the larynx. Laryngeal cancer affects more men than women, and important causative factors are smoking and excessive alcohol intake. Patients who continue to smoke and drink alcohol during treatment tend to have a decreased chance of cure and an increased risk of a second cancer. Human papilloma virus (HPV) has also been implicated in some tumors.

Pathologically the principal histology is SCC; these may be keratinizing or non-keratinizing, well or poorly differentiated. The majority of glottic tumors arise in the anterior portion of the vocal cord, with frequent involvement of the anterior commissure.

## Staging

It is important to obtain the most accurate clinical staging for these tumors, as this will ultimately affect the management of the patient. Clinical examination, followed by direct or indirect laryngoscopy, is essential. Biopsy will provide information about the grade of the tumor, and computed tomography (CT) or magnetic resonance imaging (MRI) will also help diagnose the extent of tumor spread.

TNM definitions and stage groups for laryngeal carcinoma are given in Box 6.4 and Table 6.3.

## Treatment

Superficial tumors confined to the larynx without fixation or lymphatic spread can be cured by either radiotherapy or surgery. Because true glottic tumors have very little chance of spreading lymphatically, there is no need to include the cervical lymph node chain in a radiotherapy treatment field, which usually includes the whole of the larynx. Small tumors confined to the cord may also be treated successfully with a variety of surgical techniques such as cordectomy and laser microsurgery. The overriding factor in choice of treatment is likelihood of success while maintaining

---

**Box 6.4**   Laryngeal carcinoma—TNM definitions

**Primary tumor (T)**
- TX: Primary tumor cannot be assessed
- T0: No evidence of primary tumor
- Tis: Carcinoma in situ

*Supraglottis*
- T1: Tumor limited to one subsite of supraglottis with normal vocal cord mobility
- T2: Tumor invades mucosa of more than one adjacent subsite of supraglottis or glottis or region outside the supraglottis (e.g. mucosa of base of tongue, vallecula, medial wall of pyriform sinus) without fixation of the larynx
- T3: Tumor limited to larynx with vocal cord fixation and/or invades any of the following: postcricoid area, pre-epiglottic tissues, paraglottic space, and/or minor thyroid cartilage erosion (e.g. inner cortex)
- T4a: Tumor invades through the thyroid cartilage, and/or invades tissues beyond the larynx (e.g. trachea, soft tissues of the neck, including deep extrinsic muscles of the tongue, strap muscles, thyroid, and/or esophagus)
- T4b: Tumor invades prevertebral space, encases carotid artery, or invades mediastinal structures

*Glottis*
- T1: Tumor limited to vocal cord(s) (may involve anterior or posterior commissure) with normal mobility
  —T1a: Tumor limited to one vocal cord
  —T1b: Tumor involves both vocal cords
- T2: Tumor extends to supraglottis and/or subglottis, with or without impaired vocal cord mobility
- T3: Tumor limited to the larynx with vocal cord fixation and/or invades paraglottic space, and/or minor thyroid cartilage erosion (e.g., inner cortex)
- T4a: Tumor invades cricoid or thyroid cartilage and/or invades tissues beyond the larynx (e.g. trachea, soft tissues of neck, including extrinsic muscles of the tongue, strap muscles, thyroid, or esophagus)
- T4b: Tumor invades prevertebral space, encases carotid artery, or invades mediastinal structures

*Subglottis*
- T1: Tumor limited to the subglottis
- T2: Tumor extends to vocal cord(s) with normal or impaired mobility
- T3: Tumor limited to larynx with vocal cord fixation
- T4a: Tumor invades cricoid or thyroid cartilage and/or invades tissues beyond the larynx (e.g. trachea, soft tissues of neck, including deep extrinsic muscles of the tongue, strap muscles, thyroid, or esophagus)
- T4b: Tumor invades prevertebral space, encases carotid artery, or invades mediastinal structures

**Regional lymph node involvement (N)**
- NX: Regional lymph nodes cannot be assessed
- N0: No regional lymph node metastasis
- N1: Metastasis in a single ipsilateral lymph node, 3 cm or less in greatest dimension
- N2: Metastasis in a single ipsilateral lymph node, more than 3 cm but not more than 6 cm in greatest dimension, or in multiple ipsilateral lymph

*(continued)*

**Box 6.4** (*continued*)

nodes, none more than 6 cm in greatest dimension, or in bilateral or contralateral lymph nodes, none more than 6 cm in greatest dimension
  —N2a: Metastasis in a single ipsilateral lymph node more than 3 cm but not more than 6 cm in greatest dimension
  —N2b: Metastasis in multiple ipsilateral lymph nodes, none more than 6 cm in greatest dimension
  —N2c: Metastasis in bilateral or contralateral lymph nodes, none more than 6 cm in greatest dimension
- N3: Metastasis in a lymph node more than 6 cm in greatest dimension

**Distant metastasis (M)**
- MX: Distant metastasis cannot be assessed
- M0: No distant metastasis
- M1: Distant metastasis

**Table 6.3**   Laryngeal carcinoma—stage groups

| Stage | Primary tumor | Regional node involvement | Distant metastasis |
|-------|---------------|---------------------------|--------------------|
| 0 | Tis | N0 | M0 |
| I | T1 | N0 | M0 |
| II | T2 | N0 | M0 |
| III | T3 | N0 | M0 |
|  | T1 | N1 | M0 |
|  | T2 | N1 | M0 |
|  | T3 | N1 | M0 |
| IVA | T4a | N0 | M0 |
|  | T4a | N1 | M0 |
|  | T1 | N2 | M0 |
|  | T2 | N2 | M0 |
|  | T3 | N2 | M0 |
|  | T4a | N2 | M0 |
| IVB | T4b | Any N | M0 |
|  | Any T | N3 | M0 |
| IVC | Any T | Any N | M1 |

the function of the larynx. Larger, T2, or supraglottic tumors can also be treated successfully with radiotherapy. It is important to electively treat the cervical lymph node chain on both sides of the neck. For patients with cancer of the subglottis, combined modality therapy is generally preferred, although for the uncommon small lesions (stage I or stage II) radiation therapy alone may be used. Patients who continue to smoke throughout their treatment have significantly less chance of success and therefore should be encouraged to stop smoking. For later stage disease, radiotherapy may be the preferred option of treatment, with surgery available as a backup if radiotherapy is unsuccessful.

*Prognosis*

Prognosis is very much influenced by the T and N stage of the disease. Small tumors with no lymph node involvement have a very high chance of cure (75–95% 5-year survival). Locally advanced lesions with large lymph nodes respond poorly to any form of treatment and consequently have a poor prognosis. Patients treated for laryngeal cancers are at highest risk of recurrence in the first 2–3 years. Recurrences after 5 years are rare.

## THE TRACHEA, BRONCHI, AND LUNGS

The trachea or windpipe (Fig. 6.3) is a continuation of the larynx. It is lined with ciliated epithelium and is supported by C-shaped cartilaginous rings joined together posteriorly by the trachealis muscle. The C-shaped supporting structure allows the esophagus, which is posterior to the trachea, to distend into it when food is swallowed. The function of the trachea is simple but important, in that it maintains an open passageway for the flow of air to and from the lungs. The trachea bifurcates at the carina into the right and left main bronchi. Normally the right bronchus is slightly larger and more vertical than the left. The bronchi resemble the trachea in structure, with incomplete cartilaginous rings. As the bronchi enter the lungs at the hilum, the cartilaginous rings become whole and the bronchus immediately divides into secondary bronchi. The bronchi continue to divide into smaller and smaller tubes called bronchioles, and finally form alveoli where the exchange of gases occurs. It is difficult to identify when bronchus becomes lung, and therefore carcinomas of the bronchus and lung tend to be grouped together.

The lungs are cone-shaped organs that sit on top of the diaphragm and extend superiorly to a level just above the clavicles. The ribs encase the lungs for protection. Their medial edge is concave, with the left being slightly more concave to allow room for the heart. The main bronchus and the pulmonary vessels enter and leave at the hilum of the lung. Each lung is divided into lobes by

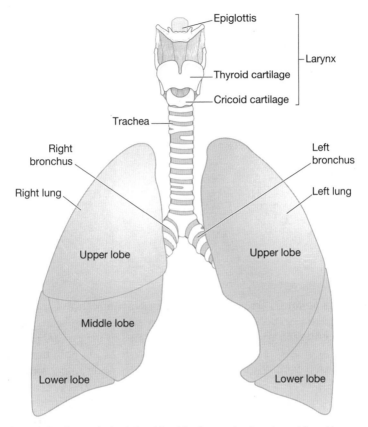

**Figure 6.3**   Anatomical relationship of the larynx, trachea, bronchi, and lungs.

fissures. The left lung is divided into two lobes, superior (upper) and inferior (lower), and the right lung is divided into three lobes, superior, middle, and inferior. The visceral pleura covers the outer surface of the lung.

## Oncology

Around 39 000 new cases of lung cancer present each year in the UK. Lung cancer continues to be the most common form of cancer in men, and the incidence in women is rising. Smoking is directly implicated in 90% of lung cancer cases, and the risk is related to the number of cigarettes smoked and the length of time since the person

---

**Box 6.5** Cellular classification of lung cancer

**Small cell carcinoma**
*Small cell (oat cell) carcinoma*
- small cell carcinoma
- mixed small cell/large cell carcinoma
- combined small cell carcinoma (small cell lung cancer combined with neoplastic squamous and/or glandular components)

**Non-small cell carcinomas**
*Squamous cell carcinoma*
- spindle cell variant

*Large cell carcinoma*
- acinar papillary
- bronchoalveolar
- solid tumor with mucin

*Adenocarcinoma*
- giant cell
- clear cell

---

started smoking. There is an increased risk of lung cancer in partners of people who smoke, indicating that passive smoking is an important causative factor. Other factors implicated in the presentation of lung cancer are environmental factors such as air pollution and industrial hazards—for example, exposure to nickel and chrome.

Lung cancer is actually two major disease processes, identified by cell type: small cell carcinoma (small or oat cell) and 'non-small cell' carcinoma (everything else). There are four main histologies: small cell (or oat cell) carcinoma, SCC (the most common), large cell carcinoma, and adenocarcinoma. Each of these has variants as indicated in Box 6.5. Adenosquamous carcinoma and undifferentiated carcinoma may also be classified as 'non-small cell' carcinoma.

Patients may present with a variety of symptoms that indicate local, lymphatic, and blood-borne spread. Local spread can involve adjacent lung tissue and give rise to respiratory symptoms such as dyspnea (shortness of breath), hemoptysis (bloodstained sputum), or infection. Invasion of adjacent organs by the tumor may occur, and pleural involvement may cause effusion. Invasion at the apex of the lung may cause pain to radiate down the arm, especially if there is involvement of the brachial nerve plexus, often referred to as Pancoast syndrome. Involvement of the recurrent laryngeal nerve may cause hoarseness. Involvement of mediastinal nodes, either directly or via lymphatic spread, may result in superior vena caval obstruction (SVCO) with associated swelling of the head and neck and engorgement of veins. SVCO is one of the few situations when emergency radiotherapy is called for. Other presenting symptoms may be the result of metastatic spread. Lung tumors tend to spread readily via the blood to brain, bone, and liver. Eighty percent of small cell tumors will present with metastatic disease.

### Staging

Staging for non-small cell lung cancer is important in the selection of appropriate treatment (see Box 6.6 and Table 6.4). Careful diagnostic evaluation of the local and metastatic extent of the tumor is crucial. Although TNM staging also applies to small cell carcinoma, the aggressive nature of small cell carcinoma and the fact that most patients present with occult metastases renders the TNM staging for this disease unemployable. Generally, small cell carcinoma is categorized into limited disease (confined to the one hemithorax), mediastinal and ipsilateral node involvement, or extensive disease with distant metastases.

### Treatment

**Small cell carcinoma**   Chemotherapy is the cornerstone of any treatment for these patients. Combination chemotherapy seems to give better results than single agent treatment but is also associated with higher levels of treatment morbidity. For patients with limited disease, local radiotherapy may be used as an adjunct to the chemotherapy. Surgery is not recommended, because of the high incidence of metastatic spread at the time of diagnosis.

**Non-small cell carcinoma**   In non-small cell lung cancer (NSCLC), results of standard treatment are poor in all but the most localized of cancers. Full assessment of the patient will determine whether or not surgery is an option. If the tumor is resectable, surgery would be the principal type of treatment. If surgery is not feasible, radical or palliative radiotherapy is the next option. Some patients may benefit from laser treatment of the tumor. NSCLC is relatively chemoresistant, and chemotherapy as a form of treatment is not usually an effective option.

Radical surgery is the only real hope of cure for patients with small localized tumors, but only about one third of patients are

**Box 6.6** Non-small cell carcinoma of the lung—TNM definitions

**Primary tumor (T)**
- TX: Primary tumor cannot be assessed, or tumor proved by the presence of malignant cells in sputum or bronchial washings, but not visualized by imaging or bronchoscopy
- T0: No evidence of primary tumor
- Tis: Carcinoma in situ
- T1: A tumor 3 cm or less in greatest dimension, surrounded by lung or visceral pleura, and without bronchoscopic evidence of invasion more proximal than the lobar bronchus[a] (i.e. not in the main bronchus)
- T2: A tumor with any of the following features of size or extent
  —more than 3 cm in greatest dimension
  —involves the main bronchus, 2 cm or more distal to the carina
  —invades the visceral pleura
  —associated with atelectasis or obstructive pneumonitis that extends to the hilar region but does not involve the entire lung
- T3:
  —A tumor of any size that directly invades any of the following: chest wall (including superior sulcus tumors), diaphragm, mediastinal pleura, parietal pericardium, or
  —tumor in the main bronchus less than 2 cm distal to the carina but without involvement of the carina, or
  —associated with atelectasis or obstructive pneumonitis of the entire lung
- T4:
  —A tumor of any size that invades any of the following: mediastinum, heart, great vessels, trachea, esophagus, vertebral body, carina, or
  —separate tumor nodules in the same lobe, or
  —tumor with a malignant pleural effusion[b]

**Regional lymph node involvement (N)**
- NX: Regional lymph nodes cannot be assessed
- N0: No regional lymph node metastasis
- N1: Metastasis to ipsilateral peribronchial and/or ipsilateral hilar lymph nodes, and intrapulmonary nodes including involvement by direct extension of the primary tumor
- N2: Metastasis to ipsilateral mediastinal and/or subcarinal lymph node(s)
- N3: Metastasis to contralateral mediastinal, contralateral hilar, ipsilateral or contralateral scalene, or supraclavicular lymph node(s)

**Distant metastasis (M)**
- MX: Distant metastasis cannot be assessed
- M0: No distant metastasis
- M1: Distant metastasis[c]

---

[a]The uncommon superficial tumor of any size with its invasive component limited to the bronchial wall, which may extend proximal to the main bronchus, is also classified T1.

[b]Most pleural effusions associated with lung cancer are due to tumor. However, there are a few patients in whom multiple cytopathologic examinations of pleural fluid are negative for tumor. In these cases, fluid is non-bloody and is not an exudate. Such patients may be further evaluated by videothoracoscopy (VATS) and direct pleural biopsies. When these elements and clinical judgment dictate that the effusion is not related to the tumor, the effusion should be excluded as a staging element and the patient should be staged as T1, T2, or T3.

[c]M1 includes separate tumor nodule(s) in a different lobe (ipsilateral or contralateral).

**Table 6.4**   Non-small cell carcinoma of the lung—stage groups

| Stage | Primary tumor | Regional node involvement | Distant metastasis |
|---|---|---|---|
| Occult carcinoma | TX | N0 | M0 |
| 0 | Tis | N0 | M0 |
| IA | T1 | N0 | M0 |
| IB | T2 | N0 | M0 |
| IIA | T1 | N1 | M0 |
| IIB | T2 | N1 | M0 |
|  | T3 | N0 | M0 |
| IIIA | T1 | N2 | M0 |
|  | T2 | N2 | M0 |
|  | T3 | N1 | M0 |
|  | T3 | N2 | M0 |
| IIIB | Any T | N3 | M0 |
|  | T4 | Any N | M0 |
| IV | Any T | Any N | M1 |

eligible. Total pneumonectomy is advisable for tumors involving the main stem bronchus, or if the tumor involves more than one lobe or the hilum. If only one lobe is involved, lobectomy may be the preferred option.

Radical radiotherapy should be considered for those patients in whom surgery is contraindicated, but only if the disease is localized. It is only suitable for a few patients. Palliative radiotherapy is helpful in relieving symptoms. Small doses can substantially improve patients' quality of life.

### Prognosis

Despite treatment, the prognosis for lung cancer in general is very poor. Surgery offers the best chance of cure for NSCLC, but overall 5-year survival is less than 50%. Only approximately 6% of patients undergoing radical radiotherapy achieve cure. The rate of survival for patients with small cell carcinoma is even worse, with few patients surviving 2 years.

## THE PLEURA

At this point it is worth mentioning the pleura. Although not part of the respiratory system, the pleural cavity plays an important role in respiration, and is host to an important form of malignant tumor. The pleural cavity consists of two layers of membrane. The parietal layer lines the inside of the ribs and the superior surface of the diaphragm and partitions the mediastinum. The visceral layer of the pleura, a separate pleural sac, covers the outer surface of the lung and encases each lung. The parietal and visceral layers are separated by a space containing a small amount of serous fluid that aids lubrication, thus allowing friction-free movement between the lungs and thoracic cavity on breathing.

Although the pleurae are not lung tissue, because of their close relationship, pleural and lung tumors are often grouped together. Malignant tumors of the pleura are primarily *mesotheliomas*. Mesothelioma is linked directly with exposure to asbestos, particularly blue asbestos; however, presentation of the disease often takes many years. At diagnosis, the tumor tends to be widespread throughout the pleural cavity. This is a direct result of transcoelomic spread throughout the serous fluid. Prognosis is difficult to determine because there is wide variation in the time before diagnosis and progression of the disease.

Localized disease is treated mainly with surgery, with extra-pleural pneumonectomy offering the best chance of recurrence-free survival. Treatment for extensive disease is rarely curative, although radiotherapy can offer palliation of symptoms.

## SELF-ASSESSMENT QUESTIONS

Answer true or false to the following. Answers are on page 244.

1. The nasopharynx extends from the base of the skull to the level of the hyoid bone.
2. The fossa of Rosenmüller is a common place for presentation of nasopharyngeal tumors.
3. Nasopharyngeal carcinoma is more common in people of Chinese origin.
4. Most pharyngeal tumors are adenocarcinomas.
5. T2 tumors of the oropharynx include a tumor larger than 4 cm in greatest dimension.
6. Smoking and alcohol intake are not associated with oropharyngeal tumors.
7. Pyriform fossa tumors make up the majority of laryngopharynx tumors.
8. Many patients with carcinoma of the laryngopharynx have cervical lymph node metastases at presentation.
9. The larynx is divided into three regions: the supraglottic, glottic, and subglottic.
10. Glottic tumors tend to present early with cervical lymph node enlargement.
11. Patients who drink and smoke while undergoing treatment for a larynx tumor have a decreased chance of cure.
12. T1 glottic tumors suggest that the vocal cords are immobile.
13. The left lung is divided into three lobes.
14. Smoking is implicated in all lung cancer cases.
15. Small cell carcinoma of the lung is usually treated with chemotherapy.
16. Non-small cell carcinoma is sometimes referred to as oat cell carcinoma.
17. Giant cell carcinoma is a variant of adenocarcinoma of the lung.
18. T1 N0 M0 would be interpreted as an early stage lung tumor.
19. Mesothelioma often spreads transcoelomically.
20. Smoking causes mesothelioma.

# The digestive system

The digestive system is concerned with the ingestion, digestion, and absorption of nutrients that can be used for metabolic processes by living cells. It is composed of numerous organs (Fig. 7.1). Some, such as the stomach and intestine, have a direct effect on the absorption of foodstuffs. Others, such as the pancreas, liver, and gallbladder, have an indirect effect and are termed accessory organs because they produce secretions which are transported to the intestines to aid the breakdown of food.

## ORAL CAVITY

The digestive system begins at the oral cavity where food first enters the digestion pathway. The oral cavity extends from the vermilion border of the lip (where the skin of the face meets the true lip) to the junction of the hard and soft palate superiorly and to the line of circumvallate papillae (taste buds) inferiorly. The oral cavity is divided into the lips, tongue, buccal (cheek) mucosa, floor of the mouth, gingiva (gums), and hard palate. The three sets of tonsils found at the back of the oral cavity where it extends into the oropharynx (Fig. 7.2) are described in Chapter 6.

Many structures within the head and neck share lymphatic drainage. An understanding of where tumors are likely to spread to is of vital importance in the management of head and neck tumors. The main routes of lymphatic drainage for this anatomic area are to the buccinator, jugulodigastric, submandibular, and

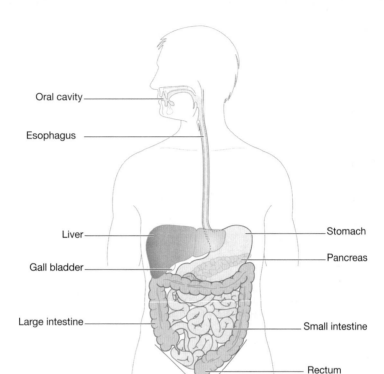

**Figure 7.1** Organs of the digestive system.

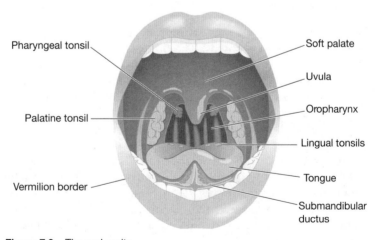

**Figure 7.2** The oral cavity.

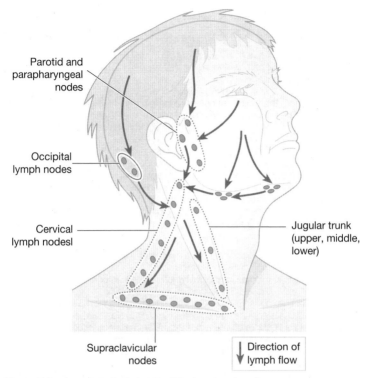

Parotid and
parapharyngeal
nodes

Occipital
lymph nodes

Cervical
lymph nodesl

Jugular trunk
(upper, middle,
lower)

Supraclavicular
nodes

Direction of
lymph flow

**Figure 7.3**  Lymph node drainage of the head and neck.

submental nodes initially (Fig. 7.3). Subsequent lymphatic drainage includes the parotid and jugular nodes, as well as the upper and lower cervical chain of nodes.

## Oncology

The oral cavity is lined with a mucous membrane composed of squamous epithelium; consequently, the majority of tumors in this area are squamous cell carcinomas (SCCs). Tobacco smoking appears to be a significant health risk for oral cavity cancer. Pipe smoking has been associated with a higher risk of lip cancer, and tobacco chewing with tumors of the buccal cavity. High-spirited alcohol is also a known risk factor, and overexposure to sunlight is implicated in lip cancer. A white furry patch on the tongue that cannot be rubbed off, called *leukoplakia*, is thought to be a pre-cancerous condition that affects the oral cavity.

---

**Box 7.1**  Staging of oral cavity cancer—TNM definitions

**Primary tumor (T)**
- TX: Primary tumor cannot be assessed
- T0: No evidence of primary tumor
- Tis: Carcinoma in situ
- T1: Tumor 2 cm or less in greatest dimension
- T2: Tumor more than 2 cm but not more than 4 cm in greatest dimension
- T3: Tumor more than 4 cm in greatest dimension
- T4: (*lip*) Tumor invades through cortical bone, inferior alveolar nerve, floor of mouth, or skin of face (i.e. chin or nose)
  - —T4a (*oral cavity*): Tumor invades adjacent structures (e.g. through cortical bone, into deep (extrinsic) muscles of tongue (genioglossus, hyoglossus, palatoglossus, and styloglossus), maxillary sinus, skin of face
  - —T4b: Tumor invades masticator space, pterygoid plates, or skull base, and/or encases internal carotid artery
  (Note: Superficial erosion alone of bone/tooth socket by gingival primary is not sufficient to classify as T4)

**Regional lymph nodes (N)**
- NX: Regional lymph nodes cannot be assessed
- N0: No regional lymph node metastasis
- N1: Metastasis in a single ipsilateral lymph node, 3 cm or less in greatest dimension
- N2: Metastasis in a single ipsilateral lymph node, more than 3 cm but not more than 6 cm in greatest dimension; or in multiple ipsilateral lymph nodes, none more than 6 cm in greatest dimension; or in bilateral or contralateral lymph nodes, none more than 6 cm in greatest dimension
  - —N2a: Metastasis in a single ipsilateral lymph node more than 3 cm but not more than 6 cm in dimension
  - —N2b: Metastasis in multiple ipsilateral lymph nodes, none more than 6 cm in greatest dimension
  - —N2c: Metastasis in bilateral or contralateral lymph nodes, none more than 6 cm in greatest dimension
- N3: Metastasis in a lymph node more than 6 cm in greatest dimension

**Distant metastasis (M)**
- MX: Distant metastasis cannot be assessed
- M0: No distant metastasis
- M1: Distant metastasis

---

*Staging*

Tumors of the oral cavity are usually classified into well differentiated, moderately differentiated, poorly differentiated, or undifferentiated (G1–G4, respectively). Staging is done using indirect or direct laryngoscopy where necessary, with clinical examination of likely nodal drainage areas on both sides of the head and neck. Box 7.1 and Table 7.1 give the TNM definitions and stage groups for oral cavity cancer.

**Table 7.1** Lip and oral cavity cancer—stage groups

| Stage | Primary tumor | Regional node involvement | Distant metastasis |
| --- | --- | --- | --- |
| 0 | Tis | N0 | M0 |
| I | T1 | N0 | M0 |
| II | T2 | N0 | M0 |
| III | T3 | N0 | M0 |
| | T1 | N1 | M0 |
| | T2 | N1 | M0 |
| | T3 | N1 | M0 |
| IVA | T4a | N0 | M0 |
| | T4a | N1 | M0 |
| | T1 | N2 | M0 |
| | T2 | N2 | M0 |
| | T3 | N2 | M0 |
| | T4a | N2 | M0 |
| IVB | T4b | Any N | M0 |
| | Any T | N3 | M0 |
| IVC | Any T | Any N | M1 |

## The lip

Lip cancers comprise approximately 25% of oral cavity tumors and are predominantly SCCs. Males are much more likely to get lip cancer, probably because of smoking. Exposure to sunlight is also implicated, and is a reason why the lower lip is often more affected than the upper lip, which generally is afforded more protection.

Interestingly, basal cell carcinoma of the lip is very rare. Where the lip is involved with this type of tumor, it is more often than not the case that a skin of face tumor has extended onto the lip. Fortunately, people tend to present early with cancer of the lip, probably for cosmetic reasons. This early presentation means that results of treatment are very good. Surgery or radiotherapy may be used either alone or in combination. Radiotherapy may involve external beam or interstitial brachytherapy.

## The oral cavity

Tumors of the oral cavity are generally SCCs and treated using either surgery or radiotherapy or a combination. One of the significant factors in choosing treatment is the anticipated functional deficit that surgery may involve. Consequently, early stage tumors tend to be treated using external beam radiotherapy. It is most important that possible routes of lymphatic spread are fully examined and, if positive, included in any treatment of the patient. This may involve block dissection of the nodes or inclusion of the lymphatic drainage in the radiotherapy treatment field. Either treatment modality offers a good chance of cure.

### The tongue

The tongue is a solid mass of skeletal muscle that is covered with a mucous membrane. Its muscles run in many directions, giving it the high maneuverability that is required in the processes of both mastication and phonation. It has a blunt root, which inserts into the back of the oral cavity, a tip, and a central body. Descriptively and oncologically, the tongue can be divided into the anterior two thirds and the posterior third, separated by the sulcus terminalis, a V-shaped line on the dorsal aspect (see Fig. 7.4). The anterior two thirds' surface is moist and covered with papillae (taste buds). Approximately 75% of all tongue tumors, the majority of which are SCCs with the occasional adenocarcinoma, arise on the anterior two thirds. Extension of the tongue outside the oral cavity means that there is good accessibility for surgical techniques. These tumors may be treated with radiotherapy or surgery, or a combination. The aim of any treatment is to offer a good chance of cure while maintaining function wherever possible. Interstitial brachytherapy in the form of iridium-192 wires may also be employed.

Posterior third tumors of the tongue warrant a different management approach. This part of the tongue comprises lymphatic tissue called the lingual tonsils. The common histology is lymphoma, most commonly non-Hodgkin lymphoma (see Ch. 2). Because these tumors are highly radiosensitive, they often receive external beam radiotherapy, which uses large fields to include the primary site and associated lymphatic drainage.

It is important to note that patients who continue to smoke while receiving radiation therapy for oral cavity tumors appear to have lower response rates and shorter survival times than those who do not.

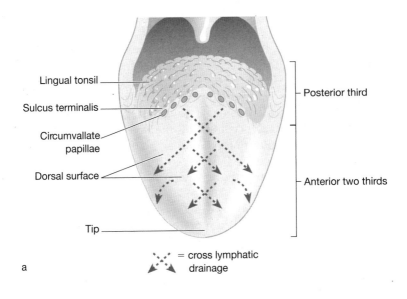

a

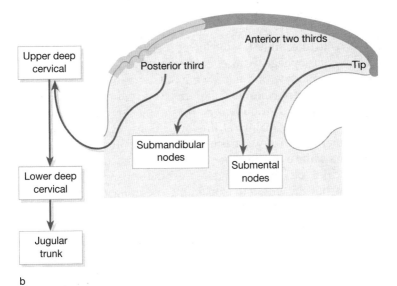

b

**Figure 7.4**   (a) Anatomy of the tongue and cross-lymphatic drainage; (b) lymphatic drainage of the tongue.

# ESOPHAGUS

The esophagus is a tube that extends from the pharynx to the stomach, allowing the passage of food. It is approximately 25 cm long and lies immediately posterior to the trachealis muscle of the trachea (a possible route of tumor spread) and anterior to the cervical and thoracic vertebrae. Flat when not in use, it is able to distend into the space occupied by the soft trachealis muscle, to accommodate a bolus of food. The esophagus has an abrasion-resistant lining surrounded by layers of striated muscle. The esophagus can conveniently be divided up into three sections: upper, middle, and lower. The cell type of the inner mucosa changes from the upper to lower regions: from squamous epithelial type in the upper third to more glandular epithelium in the lower third. The esophagus enters the stomach at the cardia through the cardiac sphincter.

## Oncology

Esophageal cancer is slightly more common in males and usually occurs in the 60–80 year age group. It is rare below 50 years of age, and tends to affect those in the lower socio-economic groups. The incidence of esophageal cancer continues to rise, and, whereas previously the majority of cancers were SCCs arising from the stratified squamous epithelium of the upper and middle thirds of the esophagus, this distribution is beginning to change. Adenocarcinomas arising mainly at the lower third region are now the predominant histology, particularly in the USA. Squamous cell carcinoma of the esophagus has been widely associated with smoking and drinking (the two together exhibit synergism), as well as poor diet, but this does not explain the rise in incidence of adenocarcinoma, which is not linked with either of these etiologic factors. The rise in incidence of Barrett's esophagus may offer a useful explanation. Long-term regurgitation of stomach contents into the lower third of the esophagus may lead to dysplastic changes that result in Barrett's esophagus, which is thought to be a high risk factor in developing adenocarcinoma of the lower esophagus.

### Staging

Staging of esophageal tumors is primarily based on the level of infiltration through the muscle layer of the esophagus. However,

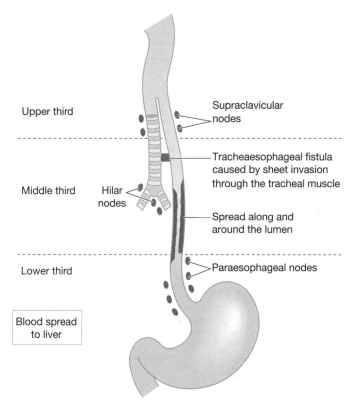

**Figure 7.5**    Possible routes of spread for esophageal tumors.

this is imprecise because modern imaging techniques, such as ultrasound and computed tomography, still cannot accurately assess the degree of infiltration. An esophageal tumor is likely to spread microscopically along and around the lumen of the esophagus (Fig. 7.5), leading to the patient's presenting with progressive dysphagia, resulting usually in massive weight loss. Patients tend to be very undernourished and dehydrated. The location of the tumor will influence the likely lymphatic spread of the tumor, with upper third tumors draining to the paratracheal and supraclavicular nodes, middle third to the hilar and mediastinal nodes, and lower third tumors draining to the paraesophageal and gastric nodes. Because the esophagus is the first part of the digestive tube proper, its blood will ultimately go to the liver, a likely route of

---

**Box 7.2** Staging of cancer of the esophagus—TNM definitions

**Primary tumor (T)**
- TX: Primary tumor cannot be assessed
- T0: No evidence of primary tumor
- Tis: Carcinoma in situ
- T1: Tumor invades lamina propria or submucosa
- T2: Tumor invades muscularis propria
- T3: Tumor invades adventitia
- T4: Tumor invades adjacent structures

**Regional lymph node involvement (N)**
- NX: Regional lymph nodes cannot be assessed
- N0: No regional lymph node metastasis
- N1: Regional lymph node metastasis

**Distant metastasis (M)**
- MX: Distant metastasis cannot be assessed
- M0: No distant metastasis
- M1: Distant metastasis

---

**Table 7.2** Esophageal cancer—stage groups

| Stage | Primary tumor | Regional lymph node involvement | Distant metastasis |
|-------|---------------|----------------------------------|--------------------|
| 0 | Tis | N0 | M0 |
| I | T1 | N0 | M0 |
| IIA | T2 | N0 | M0 |
|  | T3 | N0 | M0 |
| IIB | T1 | N1 | M0 |
|  | T2 | N1 | M0 |
| III | T3 | N1 | M0 |
|  | T4 | Any N | M0 |
| IV | Any T | Any N | M1 |

spread. Box 7.2 and Table 7.2 give TNM definitions and stage groups for cancer of the esophagus.

## Treatment

Treatment of esophageal cancer is based on whether a cure or palliation is intended. Once this decision has been established, there is a choice between surgery and radiotherapy. For early lesions, which are rare, external beam radiotherapy is the treatment choice for upper and middle third lesions, with surgery being

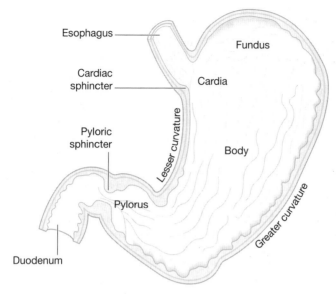

**Figure 7.6** The stomach.

reserved for lower third. High doses of radiotherapy are hard for usually emaciated older people to tolerate. Colonic transposition following total esophagectomy is also major surgery that may be difficult to tolerate. Unfortunately, results of treatment are poor for this type of cancer, with few patients surviving 5 years.

## STOMACH

The stomach lies mainly in the left upper quadrant of the abdomen between the esophagus and small intestine. It is normally J-shaped and has a greater and a lesser curvature (Fig. 7.6). The right part of the stomach lies under the liver; the left part is under the diaphragm, upon which the left lung sits. The stomach acts mainly as a storage area and is able to distend to accommodate large quantities of food. This distension occurs mainly at the superior portion of the stomach and therefore restricts the potential movement of the lungs inferiorly, giving the feeling of shortness of breath after overeating. Anatomically, the stomach is divided into various sections. The cardiac region, where the esophagus enters, is bordered by the cardiac sphincter (valve), which allows foodstuffs to pass into the stomach, but not back into the esophagus. Heartburn is caused by reflux of the acidic contents of the stomach back through this sphincter and burning of the lower esophagus. Partially digested foodstuff passes from the stomach into the small intestine via the pyloric sphincter.

The fundus of the stomach acts as a storage area and is the part which pushes upwards on the undersurface of the diaphragm. Food moves from the fundus to the body of the stomach, a central portion where food is churned and mixed with the gastric secretions. The final section is the pylorus, the distal end of the stomach which joins the duodenum via the pyloric sphincter. The mucosa of the stomach is lined with simple columnar epithelium containing large numbers of gastric glands. These glands secrete most of the gastric juice, a mucus-type fluid containing enzymes and hydrochloric acid. The stomach is a highly muscular organ with longitudinal, circular and oblique muscle fibers allowing the stomach to contract in different directions so that the food is broken up and mixed effectively. The lining of the stomach and the remainder of the digestive system contain aggregated lymphatic tissue, and local lymphatic drainage is to the gastric and splenic nodes.

## Oncology

Worldwide, cancer of the stomach is still a significant health risk, although generally the incidence is declining. The highest incidences are recorded in Japan and other east Asian countries. It is a disease that is twice as common in men, although this varies with age, and older age groups generally have a higher incidence. Several risk factors are associated with stomach cancer: *Helicobacter pylori* infection, a diet including dry salted foods, atrophic gastritis, pernicious anemia, cigarette smoking, and familial polyposis. Multiple daily rations of fruit and vegetables may have a preventive effect, along with vitamin C.

Most tumors of the stomach are adenocarcinomas (subdivided into ulcerative, polypoid, scirrhous, and superficially spreading types), with carcinoid tumors (see later), lymphomas, and leiomyosarcomas making up the rest of the histologies. Staging is determined by the extent of invasion into the muscle layer of the stomach. Spread is to the regional lymphatics, which do have a bearing on the prognosis for the patient. Unfortunately, because of the ability of the stomach to distend with minimal discomfort,

**Box 7.3**    Staging of stomach cancer—TNM definitions

**Primary tumor (T)**
- TX: Primary tumor cannot be assessed
- T0: No evidence of primary tumor
- Tis: Carcinoma in situ: intraepithelial tumor without invasion of the lamina propria
- T1: Tumor invades lamina propria or submucosa
- T2: Tumor invades the muscularis propria or the subserosa[a]
  —T2a Tumor invades muscularis propria
  —T2b Tumor invades subserosa
- T3: Tumor penetrates the serosa (visceral peritoneum) without invading adjacent structures[b,c]
- T4: Tumor invades adjacent structures[b,c]

**Regional lymph node involvement (N)**
- NX: Regional lymph node(s) cannot be assessed
- N0: No regional lymph node metastasis
- N1: Metastasis in 1 to 6 regional lymph nodes
- N2: Metastasis in 7 to 15 regional lymph nodes
- N3: Metastasis in more than 15 regional lymph nodes

**Distant metastasis (M)**
- MX: Distant metastasis cannot be assessed
- M0: No distant metastasis
- M1: Distant metastasis

[a] A tumor may penetrate the muscularis propria with extension into the gastrocolic or gastrohepatic ligaments, or into the greater or lesser omentum, without perforation of the visceral peritoneum covering these structures. In this case, the tumor is classified T2. If there is perforation of the visceral peritoneum covering the gastric ligaments or the omentum, the tumor should be classified T3.
[b] The adjacent structures of the stomach include the spleen, transverse colon, liver, diaphragm, pancreas, abdominal wall, adrenal gland, kidney, small intestine, and retroperitoneum.
[c] Intramural extension to the duodenum or esophagus is classified by the depth of the greatest invasion in any of these sites, including the stomach.

patients tend to present at late stages, with distant metastases already present, leading to an overall poor prognosis.

### Staging

Box 7.3 and Table 7.3 show TNM definitions and stage groups for stomach cancer.

### Treatment

Due to the late presentation, very few patients are eligible for radical surgery, which represents the best chance of cure. However,

**Table 7.3** Stomach cancer—stage groups

| Stage | Primary tumor | Regional node involvement | Distant metastasis |
|---|---|---|---|
| 0 | Tis | N0 | M0 |
| IA | T1 | N0 | M0 |
| IB | T1 | N1 | M0 |
| | T2a/b | N0 | M0 |
| II | T1 | N2 | M0 |
| | T2a/b | N1 | M0 |
| | T3 | N0 | M0 |
| IIIA | T2a/b | N2 | M0 |
| | T3 | N1 | M0 |
| | T4 | N0 | M0 |
| IIIB | T3 | N2 | M0 |
| IV | T4 | N1–3 | M0 |
| | T1–3 | N3 | M0 |
| | Any T | Any N | M1 |

partial gastrectomy and laser therapy play an important role in palliation of symptoms. Because of the radiosensitive nature of the stomach mucosa, radiotherapy can only be tolerated in small doses, and it therefore tends to be reserved for palliative rather than curative treatment. Chemotherapy, alone or in combination with radiotherapy, also has shown little efficacy, although clinical trials continue.

## SMALL INTESTINE

The small intestine (or small bowel) is approximately 6.5 meters long and consists of the duodenum (25 cm), the jejunum (2.5 m) and the ileum (3.6 m). Its coiled loops fill most of the abdominal cavity. The duodenum is the uppermost section, and is a continuation from the pylorus of the stomach. It is shaped like a letter C, surrounds the head of the pancreas, and receives the common bile duct (from the gallbladder and liver) and the pancreatic duct at a small raised area called the hepatopancreatic ampulla (ampulla of Vater). The mucosal layer is epithelial and is lined with many glands which secrete intestinal juice, although some cells are specialized and secrete mucus (goblet cells). Other cells, called enteroendocrine cells, have a more endocrine function and produce hormones that stimulate the secretion of bicarbonated pancreatic juice to balance the intestinal pH against the effect of acidic chyme from the stomach. Enterochromaffin cells, a particular type of enteroendocrine cell, secrete serotonin, and may develop into a particular type of cancer called a carcinoid tumor (see later) within the small intestine. Scattered throughout the mucous membrane are solitary lymphatic nodules, most numerous in the lower part of the ileum. These may be joined together to form aggregated lymphatic nodules (Peyer's patches), which protect the intestines from ingested microbes and dirt. The main purpose of the small intestine is to absorb the nutrients from food. In order to do this, it has a rich blood supply. All blood from this part of the body is transported directly to the liver as part of the hepatic circulation, so liver metastasis is a common form of spread for intestinal cancer.

## Oncology

Cancer of the small intestine accounts for only a small percentage of gastrointestinal malignancies (1–2%). Different histologies tend to be present in the various parts of the small intestine, with adenocarcinoma being the main tumor type associated with the duodenum and first part of the jejunum. Lymphomas are rare in this section, but are relatively common in the ileum, along with carcinoid tumors. Rarely, leiomyosarcomas can also be found in the small intestine. Patients may present with a variety of symptoms, mainly due to obstruction, with a sense of abdominal discomfort. The length of the small intestine, along with the rich blood supply, often means that patients present with late stage disease. Curability is directly associated with the resectability of the tumor and its histology. Patients with leiomyosarcoma generally fare better than those with adenocarcinoma. Surgery is the main form of curative treatment available, with radiotherapy and chemotherapy offering little chance of cure. Box 7.4 and Table 7.4 show TNM definitions for staging cancer of the small intestine.

## LARGE INTESTINE

The large intestine (or large bowel) (Fig. 7.7) is about 1.5 meters long. It is continuous with the ileum where it becomes the cecum. The cecum is continuous upwards with the ascending colon, which turns sharply towards midline at the hepatic flexure to become the transverse colon. This in turn is deflected downwards

**Box 7.4** Staging of cancer of the small intestine—TNM definitions

**Primary tumor (T)**
- TX: Primary tumor cannot be assessed
- T0: No evidence of primary tumor
- Tis: Carcinoma in situ
- T1: Tumor invades lamina propria or submucosa
- T2: Tumor invades muscularis propria
- T3: Tumor invades through the muscularis propria into the subserosa or into the non-peritonealized perimuscular tissue (mesentery or retroperitoneum) with extension 2 cm or less[a]
- T4: Tumor perforates the visceral peritoneum or directly invades other organs or structures (includes other loops of small intestine, mesentery, or retroperitoneum more than 2 cm, and abdominal wall by way of serosa; for duodenum only, invasion of pancreas)

**Regional lymph node involvement (N)**
- NX: Regional lymph nodes cannot be assessed
- N0: No regional lymph node metastasis
- N1: Regional lymph node metastasis

**Distant metastasis (M)**
- MX: Distant metastasis cannot be assessed
- M0: No distant metastasis
- M1: Distant metastasis

[a] The non-peritonealized perimuscular tissue is: for jejunum and ileum, part of the mesentery; for duodenum, in areas where serosa is lacking, part of the retroperitoneum.

**Table 7.4** Cancer of the small intestine—stage groups

| Stage | Primary tumor | Regional node involvement | Distant metastasis |
|-------|---------------|---------------------------|--------------------|
| 0 | Tis | N0 | M0 |
| I | T1 | N0 | M0 |
|   | T2 | N0 | M0 |
| II | T3 | N0 | M0 |
|   | T4 | N0 | M0 |
| III | Any T | N1 | M0 |
| IV | Any T | Any N | M1 |

by the spleen at the splenic flexure. This downward segment is called the descending colon. Onwards, the colon forms an S-shaped curve known as the sigmoid colon, before terminating at the rectum and the anus. The large intestine is lined with columnar epithelium and mucus-secreting goblet cells. Its primary function is to absorb water.

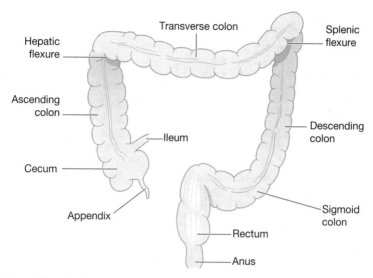

**Figure 7.7**   The large intestine.

## Oncology

Cancer of the large intestine, termed colorectal cancer, affects a significant number of people in developed countries. It is the second most common cancer in the USA. In the UK, colorectal cancer is the second most common form of cancer in women and the third most common in men. The male to female ratio is approximately 1.5:1. Adenocarcinomas are the most common type, constituting approximately 90% of cases, with carcinoid tumors and leiomyosarcomas making up the rest. The greatest proportion of cases occurs in the sigmoid colon, followed closely by the rectum and the cecum areas. A large proportion of colorectal cancers may be associated with high fat diet. Notably, incidence is much lower in parts of the world where high fiber diets are the norm, such as India. Physical activity resulting in increased peristaltic activity, and high fiber diets, tend to decrease stool transit time. This possibly limits the time any carcinogens remain in the system and is therefore associated with reduced risk of developing colon cancer. Patients with a history of benign polyps are at greater risk of developing colorectal cancer. Generally, mortality rates are decreasing in developed countries, suggesting that treatment is becoming more effective. However, because there is still a significant

---

**Box 7.5** Staging for colorectal cancer—TNM definitions

**Primary tumor (T)**
- TX: Primary tumor cannot be assessed
- T0: No evidence of primary tumor
- Tis: Carcinoma in situ: intraepithelial or invasion of lamina propria[a]
- T1: Tumor invades the submucosa
- T2: Tumor invades muscularis propria
- T3: Tumor invades through the muscularis propria into the subserosa, or into non-peritonealized pericolic or perirectal tissues
- T4: Tumor directly invades other organs or structures, and/or perforates visceral peritoneum[b,c]

**Regional lymph node involvement (N)**
- NX: Regional lymph nodes cannot be assessed
- N0: No regional lymph node metastasis
- N1: Metastases in 1 to 3 regional lymph nodes
- N2: Metastases 4 or more regional lymph nodes

**Distant metastasis (M)**
- MX: Distant metastasis cannot be assessed
- M0: No distant metastasis
- M1: Distant metastasis

[a] Tis includes cancer cells confined within the glandular basement membrane (intraepithelial) or lamina propria (intramucosal) with no extension through the muscularis mucosa into the submucosa.
[b] Direct invasion in T4 includes invasion of other segments of the colorectum by way of the serosa; for example, invasion of the sigmoid colon by a carcinoma of the cecum.
[c] Tumor that is adherent to other organs or structures, macroscopically, is classified T4. However, if no tumor is present in the adhesion, microscopically, the classification should be pT3. V and L substaging should be used to identify the presence or absence of vascular or lymphatic invasion.

---

health risk, some authorities advocate regular colonic screening for people over 50 years of age, as the incidence of colorectal cancer increases with age.

### Staging

Staging for colorectal cancer is defined by the extent of infiltration into the mucosa and muscle, and by lymph node involvement, both of which have a significant bearing on prognosis (see Box 7.5 and Table 7.5).

### Treatment

Surgery remains the cornerstone of treatment and can be curable for early stage disease. Unfortunately, modern imaging techniques

**Table 7.5**   Colorectal cancer—stage groups for TNM classification and Dukes staging system

| TNM stage | Primary tumor | Regional node involvement | Distant metastasis | Dukes stage |
|---|---|---|---|---|
| 0 | Tis | N0 | M0 | – |
| I | T1 | N0 | M0 | A |
|   | T2 | N0 | M0 | A |
| IIA | T3 | N0 | M0 | B |
| IIB | T4 | N0 | M0 | B |
| IIIA | T1–T2 | N1 | M0 | C |
| IIIB | T3–T4 | N1 | M0 | C |
| IIIC | Any T | N2 | M0 | C |
| IV | Any T | Any N | M1 | – |

cannot always accurately assess the extent of the disease and associated lymphatic involvement. Because of the vascular nature of the colon, many patients have blood-borne spread to the liver on presentation. A common problem with surgery is inadequate resection of the tumor, resulting in recurrence of the tumor. Radiation therapy and chemotherapy (5-fluorouracil) may also be used in combination.

# Anal cancer

The anal canal is approximately 4 cm long and extends from the rectum to the anal orifice. The lower half is lined by squamous epithelium and the upper half by columnar epithelium. Anal cancer is an uncommon malignancy, and the main histology is SCC in the lower half, with the occasional adenocarcinoma in the upper half and some melanomas. Overall, the incidence of anal cancer is increasing. Individuals with the human papilloma virus are at increased risk, along with male homosexuals. The main presenting symptoms are bleeding, pain, and itching, which can often be confused with those of hemorrhoids. Box 7.6 and Table 7.6 give TNM definitions and stage groups for anal cancer.

## *Treatment*

Small tumors may be resected locally, while radiotherapy offers a good chance of cure for larger tumors. Brachytherapy may be used in order to increase the dose to the immediate anal area.

---

**Box 7.6** Staging of anal cancer—TNM definitions

**Primary tumor (T)**
- TX: Primary tumor cannot be assessed
- T0: No evidence of primary tumor
- Tis: Carcinoma in situ
- T1: Tumor 2 cm or less in greatest dimension
- T2: Tumor more than 2 cm but not more than 5 cm in greatest dimension
- T3: Tumor more than 5 cm in greatest dimension
- T4: Tumor of any size that invades adjacent organ(s), e.g. vagina, urethra, bladder[a]

**Regional lymph node involvement (N)**
- NX: Regional lymph nodes cannot be assessed
- N0: No regional lymph node metastasis
- N1: Metastasis in perirectal lymph node(s)
- N2: Metastasis in unilateral internal iliac and/or inguinal lymph node(s)
- N3: Metastasis in perirectal and inguinal lymph nodes and/or bilateral internal iliac and/or inguinal lymph nodes

**Distant metastasis (M)**
- MX: Distant metastasis cannot be assessed
- M0: No distant metastasis
- M1: Distant metastasis

---

[a] Direct invasion of the rectal wall, perirectal skin, subcutaneous tissue or the sphincter muscle(s) is not classified as T4.

---

**Table 7.6** Anal cancer—stage groups

| Stage | Primary tumor | Regional node involvement | Distant metastasis |
|---|---|---|---|
| 0 | Tis | N0 | M0 |
| I | T1 | N0 | M0 |
| II | T2 | N0 | M0 |
| | T3 | N0 | M0 |
| IIIA | T1 | N1 | M0 |
| | T2 | N1 | M0 |
| | T3 | N1 | M0 |
| | T4 | N0 | M0 |
| IIIB | T4 | N1 | M0 |
| | Any T | N2 | M0 |
| | Any T | N3 | M0 |
| | Any T | Any N | M1 |

High doses of radiation may cause problems with fibrosis of the anal canal and/or sphincter in the long term. Concurrent chemotherapy has been shown to improve survival rates in selected patients.

# LIVER, PANCREAS, AND GALLBLADDER

The liver, pancreas, and gallbladder are accessory organs of the digestive system. They produce secretions that are transported to the small intestine via a series of ducts to aid in the breakdown of foodstuffs. Bile, produced by hepatocytes in the liver, is stored in the gallbladder. When needed, it flows to the small intestine via the common bile duct. Just before entering the duodenum, the common bile duct combines with the pancreatic duct, which brings bicarbonated pancreatic juice to the small intestine. Both join the duodenum at the hepatopancreatic ampulla (ampulla of Vater).

## Liver

The liver is the largest gland in the body and lies under the diaphragm. It extends from the right side across the midline to the stomach. The liver is divided into the right and left lobes (Fig. 7.8). The right lobe is further subdivided into the right lobe proper, the caudate lobe and the quadrate lobe. Each lobe is divided into hepatic lobules, which are roughly hexagonal in shape. Each lobule is made up of epithelial cells called hepatocytes (true liver cells), arranged in irregular columns around a central vein. Blood sinusoids, which are partly lined with stellate reticuloendothelial cells (Kupffer cells), run between the columns. The Kupffer cells destroy worn-out red and white blood cells. Surrounding the liver cells are bile canaliculi, which collect bile produced by the hepatocytes and transfer it to the right and left hepatic ducts. The liver receives blood from two sources: the hepatic artery (a direct branch of the aorta), and the hepatic portal vein, which carries blood rich in nutrients, toxins, and possibly drugs from the digestive tract. This blood is conveyed to the lobules, and the nutrients and oxygen are taken up by the hepatocytes. The hepatocytes in turn secrete their products, which may be needed by other cells, back into the blood. Each lobule is supplied with an abundance of blood, making the liver an extremely vascular organ. Because all the blood from the digestive tract goes first to the liver, it is a common site for metastases.

Primary liver tumors are rare and potentially curable with surgical resection. There are two main histologies: hepatocellular carcinoma and cholangiosarcoma. However, metastases to the liver

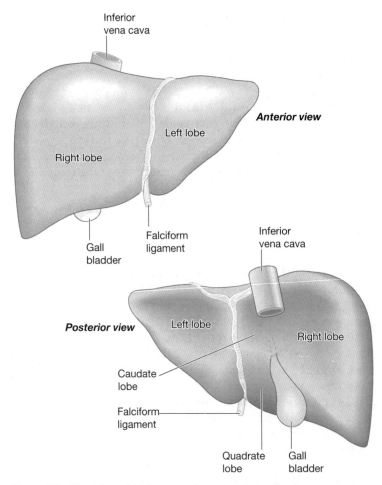

**Figure 7.8** The lobes of the liver, anterior and posterior views.

remain the most common tumor in the liver. Hepatoblastoma may also occur in children. While hepatitis B and hepatitis C are associated with most cases of hepatocellular carcinoma, cirrhosis is also found in a large percentage of cases. Raised alfa-fetoprotein levels can indicate the presence of hepatocellular carcinoma and can be used as a tumor marker. Most patients present with multi-focal disease, making surgical cure difficult to achieve. However, surgery offers the main chance of cure. Box 7.7 and Table 7.7 give the TNM definitions and stage groups for liver cancer.

---

**Box 7.7**   Staging of liver cancer—TNM definitions

**Primary tumor (T)**
- TX: Primary tumor cannot be assessed
- T0: No evidence of primary tumor
- T1: Solitary tumor without vascular invasion
- T2: Solitary tumor with vascular invasion or multiple tumors, none more than 5 cm in greatest dimension
- T3: Multiple tumors more than 5 cm or tumor involving a major branch of the portal or hepatic vein(s)
- T4: Tumor(s) with direct invasion of adjacent organs other than the gallbladder or with perforation of visceral peritoneum

**Regional lymph node involvement (N)**
- NX: Regional lymph nodes cannot be assessed
- N0: No regional lymph node metastasis
- N1: Regional lymph node metastasis

**Distant metastasis (M)**
- MX: Distant metastasis cannot be assessed
- M0: No distant metastasis
- M1: Distant metastasis

---

**Table 7.7**   Liver cancer—stage groups

| Stage | Primary tumor | Regional node involvement | Distant metastasis |
|-------|---------------|---------------------------|--------------------|
| I | T1 | N0 | M0 |
| II | T2 | N0 | M0 |
| IIIA | T3 | N0 | M0 |
| IIIB | T4 | N0 | M0 |
| IIIC | Any T | N1 | M0 |
| IV | Any T | Any N | M1 |

# Pancreas

The pancreas (Fig. 7.9) lies behind the stomach in the C-shaped loop of the duodenum in direct contact with the stomach and spleen. Major blood vessels, such as the mesenteric artery and veins, pass close to the body of the pancreas. Microscopically, the pancreas is composed of a large number of lobules surrounded by fatty tissue. Each lobule is composed of glandular epithelium lined with many specialized cells that produce pancreatic secretions. Of these cells, 1% are called pancreatic islets and the other 99% are

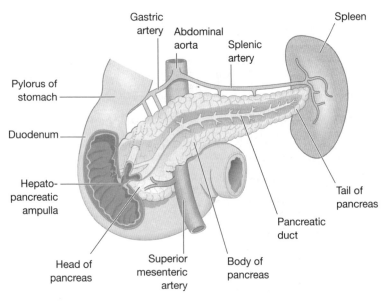

**Figure 7.9** Relational anatomy of the pancreas.

acinic cells. The pancreatic islets are the endocrine portion of the pancreas and secrete glucagon, insulin, and somatostatin. The acinic cells secrete pancreatic juice to aid the digestive process. Pancreatic juice is secreted into the pancreatic duct which transports the juice to the duodenum via the hepatopancreatic ampulla (ampulla of Vater). Shortly before this ampulla, the pancreatic duct is joined by the common bile duct from the liver and gallbladder. Because of the proximity of so many organs, it is common for a pancreatic cancer to invade one or more of these structures. This makes pancreatic cancer very difficult to cure.

Pancreatic cancer ranks as the tenth and eleventh most common cancers in males and females of the UK, respectively. It ranks as the fifth most common cancer in the USA. Because of the poor prognosis associated with the disease, pancreatic cancer constitutes a significant health risk. Men are more likely to get the disease, although the male to female ratio is becoming more even. This may be due to the fact that smoking is a high risk factor for pancreatic cancer. Mortality rates tend to mirror the incidence rates, with patients rarely surviving a year, but, fortunately, the incidence of the disease worldwide is declining. Most pancreatic

---

**Box 7.8**    Staging of cancer of the exocrine pancreas—TNM definitions

**Primary tumor (T)**
- TX: Primary tumor cannot be assessed
- T0: No evidence of primary tumor
- Tis: Carcinoma in situ
- T1: Tumor limited to the pancreas, 2 cm or less in greatest dimension
- T2: Tumor limited to the pancreas, more than 2 cm in greatest dimension
- T3: Tumor extends beyond the pancreas but without involvement of the celiac axis or the superior mesenteric artery
- T4: Tumor involves the celiac axis or the superior mesenteric artery (unresectable primary tumor)

**Regional lymph node involvement (N)**
- NX: Regional lymph nodes cannot be assessed
- N0: No regional lymph node metastasis
- N1: Regional lymph node metastasis

**Distant metastasis (M)**
- MX: Distant metastasis cannot be assessed
- M0: No distant metastasis
- M1: Distant metastasis

---

**Table 7.8**    Pancreatic cancer—stage groups

| Stage | Primary tumor | Regional node involvement | Distant metastasis |
|-------|---------------|---------------------------|--------------------|
| 0     | Tis           | N0                        | M0                 |
| IA    | T1            | N0                        | M0                 |
| IB    | T2            | N0                        | M0                 |
| IIA   | T3            | N0                        | M0                 |
| IIB   | T1            | N1                        | M0                 |
|       | T2            | N1                        | M0                 |
|       | T3            | N1                        | M0                 |
| III   | T4            | Any N                     | M0                 |
| IV    | Any T         | Any N                     | M1                 |

tumors are of ductal type (adenocarcinomas), but other variants may occur, such as acinar cell carcinoma, papillary mucinous carcinoma, signet ring carcinoma, adenosquamous carcinoma, undifferentiated carcinoma, mucinous carcinoma, and giant cell carcinoma. Survival for patients with pancreatic cancer is poor, with surgery offering the best chance of disease-free survival. Box 7.8 and Table 7.8 give TNM definitions and stage groups for cancer of the exocrine pancreas.

The endocrine portion of the pancreas consists of alfa (A) cells, beta (B) cells, delta (D) cells, and F cells. Table 7.9 shows the hormones secreted by these cells, and the tumors associated with

**Table 7.9**   Cells of the endocrine pancreas with associated hormones and tumors

| Cell type | Hormone | Hormone action | Tumor type |
|---|---|---|---|
| Alfa | Glucagon | Raises blood glucose levels by stimulating hepatocytes | Glucagonoma |
| Beta | Insulin | Decreases blood glucose levels by stimulating body cells to take up glucose from the blood | Insulinoma |
| Delta | Somatostatin | Inhibits secretion of glucagon and insulin and slows GI absorption process | Somatostatinoma, gastrinoma |
| F | Polypeptide | Inhibits the secretion of somatostatin | None, although does produce multiple hormone syndromes |

them. Surgery remains the best chance of cure with early stage disease often quite curable in contrast to adenocarcinoma of the exocrine pancreas. There is no TNM staging classification for endocrine cancers of the pancreas.

# Gallbladder

The gallbladder is a pear-shaped organ that lies on the undersurface of the liver. Its function is to store bile and secrete it into the duodenum via the common bile duct when influenced by the amount of fat in the intestine. Bile is an emulsifier; that is, it breaks down fat in order for the body to process it more easily. Gallbladder cancer is uncommon and tends to be associated with gallstones. Many patients are found to have cancer on routine removal of the gallbladder as a remedy for gallstones. This leads to cure with no further treatment required. The majority of tumors of the gallbladder are adenocarcinomas of various subtypes: signet ring cell, clear cell, colloid, small (oat) cell, and others. Gallbladder cancer that has penetrated the muscularis and serosa is curable in fewer than 5% of patients. Box 7.9 and Table 7.10 show TNM definitions and stage groups for cancer of the gallbladder.

# CARCINOID TUMORS

As mentioned earlier, carcinoid tumors can also occur in the digestive tract. They occur in enteroendocrine cells that are dispersed

**Box 7.9** Staging for cancer of the gallbladder—TNM definitions

**Primary tumor (T)**
- TX: Primary tumor cannot be assessed
- T0: No evidence of primary tumor
- Tis: Carcinoma in situ
- T1: Tumor invades lamina propria or muscle layer
  —T1a: Tumor invades lamina propria
  —T1b: Tumor invades muscle layer
- T2: Tumor invades perimuscular connective tissue; no extension beyond serosa or into liver
- T3: Tumor perforates the serosa (visceral peritoneum) and/or directly invades the liver and/or one other adjacent organ or structure, such as the stomach, duodenum, colon, or pancreas, omentum, or extrahepatic bile ducts
- T4: Tumor invades main portal vein or hepatic artery or invades multiple extrahepatic organs or structures

**Regional lymph node involvement (N)**
- NX: Regional lymph nodes cannot be assessed
- N0: No regional lymph node metastasis
- N1: Regional lymph node metastasis

**Distant metastasis (M)**
- MX: Distant metastasis cannot be assessed
- M0: No distant metastasis
- M1: Distant metastasis

**Table 7.10** Cancer of the gallbladder—stage groups

| Stage | Primary tumor | Regional node involvement | Distant metastasis |
|-------|---------------|---------------------------|--------------------|
| 0 | Tis | N0 | M0 |
| IA | T1 | N0 | M0 |
| IB | T2 | N0 | M0 |
| IIA | T3 | N0 | M0 |
| IIB | T1 | N1 | M0 |
|  | T2 | N1 | M0 |
|  | T3 | N1 | M0 |
| III | T4 | Any N | M0 |
| IV | Any T | Any N | M1 |

throughout the stomach and small and large intestines. These specialized cells are responsible for secreting hormones such as gastrin (stomach), cholecystokinin (small intestine) and secretin (small intestine). They play a role in stimulating the organs of the digestive system to generate secretions that aid the digestive process.

Carcinoid tumors are classified as *neuroendocrine tumors* and are often asymptomatic, mainly because of their slow-growing nature. They can occur anywhere where enteroendocrine cells are found, but the most common sites are the appendix, small bowel, and rectum. Patients with carcinoid tumors may present with carcinoid syndrome, typically with flushing, diarrhea, and abdominal cramps. *Carcinoid syndrome* is caused by oversecretion of serotonin by the affected cells. Surgical removal of the affected site offers a good chance of cure for localized disease. Radiotherapy and chemotherapy are largely ineffective.

## SELF-ASSESSMENT QUESTIONS

Answer true or false to the following. Answers are on page 244.

1. Pancreas, gallbladder, and liver are termed accessory organs of the digestive system.
2. Most tumors of the lip are basal cell carcinomas.
3. Most tumors of the tongue occur in the posterior third region.
4. Lymphomas are the primary histology in the posterior third of the tongue.
5. The esophagus is lined entirely with squamous epithelium.
6. Smoking and drinking are main causative factors for squamous cell carcinoma of the esophagus.
7. Staging of esophageal cancer is based on the level of infiltration through the muscle layer of the esophagus.
8. The stomach is lined with glandular epithelium.
9. Squamous cell carcinoma is the predominant tumor of the stomach.
10. The order of sections of the small intestine (in the direction of the digestive process) is ileum, jejunum, duodenum.
11. The lining of the small intestine includes aggregated lymphatic tissue.
12. Lymphomas occur mainly in the ileum section of the small intestine.
13. Adenocarcinomas make up about 90% of cases of colorectal cancer.
14. Colorectal cancer is associated with a high fiber diet.
15. The staging of colorectal cancer is based on the level of infiltration of the muscle layer.
16. The staging of anal cancer is based on the size of the primary tumor.
17. Metastases are the most common primary liver tumor.
18. The pancreas is both an endocrine and an exocrine gland.
19. Insulinoma is a typical tumor which affects the delta cells of the pancreas.
20. Carcinoid tumors arise from the enteroendocrine portion of the gastrointestinal tract.

# The urinary system

The urinary system consists of two kidneys, two ureters, one urinary bladder and one urethra.

## THE KIDNEYS AND URETERS

The kidneys are situated behind the peritoneum (retroperitoneal) on the posterior abdominal wall (Fig. 8.1). They are approximately 9 cm long and 6 cm wide and are oriented so that the upper

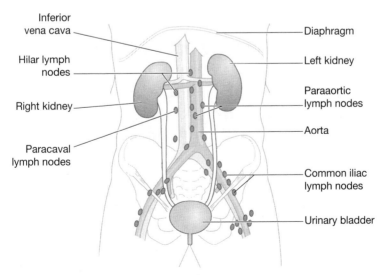

**Figure 8.1**    Relational anatomy of the kidneys, showing regional lymphatic nodes.

lobe is closer to midline. Normal kidneys have a shiny reddish-brown appearance. Their function is to regulate the volume and composition of blood in the body by removing waste materials. They cleanse the plasma, and adjust the salt and pH content. The resultant waste product is called urine. Adults normally excrete 1–1.5 liters of urine per day. Once produced, the urine is conveyed, via the ureters, to the urinary bladder where it is stored prior to excretion via the urethra.

The kidney is divided into an outer cortex and inner medulla section (Fig. 8.2). Within the medulla are 5–14 striated triangular structures called renal pyramids. The cortex extends between these pyramids, forming renal columns. The cortex and the pyramids constitute the renal parenchyma, that is, the functional part of the kidney. The *renal parenchyma* consists of millions of *nephrons* with their associated collecting ducts and blood supply. The nephrons filter the blood and ultimately produce the urine.

The urine is conveyed via the collecting tubules into the central part of the kidney, called the renal pelvis, which is typically whitish-gray in appearance. Interestingly, the cells lining the renal pelvis are transitional epithelial cells. The difference in the

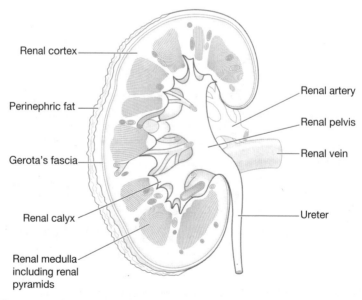

**Figure 8.2** Coronal section through the kidney.

functions of the renal parenchyma and the renal pelvis results in different malignant histologies (see below). The kidney parenchyma is surrounded by a tough renal capsule which itself is enveloped by a layer of fatty tissue called perinephric fat. Between the kidney and the psoas muscle and the lumbar spine is a band of connective tissue referred to as Gerota's fascia, an important landmark when considering advanced stages of renal carcinoma (see staging).

Lymphatically, the kidneys drain into the lymph nodes medial to the hilum (renal hilar nodes) and to the nodes surrounding the aorta (para-aortic) and inferior vena cava (paracaval). All regional lymph nodes of the kidney are retroperitoneal.

## Oncology

Carcinoma of the kidney accounts for approximately 2% of all cancers. Of these, 85% are of the kidney parenchyma (renal cell carcinomas, RCCs) and 15% are of the renal pelvis (transitional cell carcinomas). There are three basic pathologies:

- RCC: adenocarcinomas, the most common subtypes being clear cell and granular cell
- renal pelvis carcinoma: transitional cell or urothelial carcinomas
- Wilms' tumor: childhood malignancy.

### Renal cell carcinoma (RCC)

RCC is the most common of the renal malignancies. They are also known as adenocarcinomas (an older term is hypernephroma) and may be separated into clear cell and granular cell carcinomas. The male to female ratio is approximately 2:1. Presentation is most common between the ages of 60 and 70 years. The cause of this type of cancer is relatively unknown, but it is associated with smoking and intake of alcohol. RCCs predominantly arise in the epithelial lining of the proximal convoluted tubule of the nephron.

**Staging** Staging of RCC is based on the degree of spread within, and more importantly beyond, the kidney. Although involvement of blood vessels such as the vena cava is generally associated with poor prognosis, this may not be the case for disease otherwise confined to the kidney. RCCs have a tendency to metastasize to other parts of the body, principally lung, mainly via the bloodstream rather than

---

**Box 8.1**  Staging of RCC—TNM definitions

**Primary tumor (T)**
- TX: Primary tumor cannot be assessed
- T0: No evidence of primary tumor
- T1: Tumor 7 cm or less in greatest dimension, limited to the kidney
  —T1a: Tumor 4 cm or less in greatest dimension, limited to the kidney
  —T1b: Tumor more than 4 cm but not more than 7 cm in greatest dimension, limited to the kidney
- T2: Tumor more than 7 cm in greatest dimension, limited to the kidney
- T3: Tumor extends into major veins or invades adrenal gland or perinephric tissues but not beyond Gerota's fascia
  —T3a: Tumor directly invades adrenal gland or perirenal and/or renal sinus fat but not beyond Gerota's fascia
  —T3b: Tumor grossly extends into the renal vein or its segmental (muscle-containing) branches, or vena cava below the diaphragm
  —T3c: Tumor grossly extends into vena cava above diaphragm or invades the wall of the vena cava
- T4: Tumor invades beyond Gerota's fascia

**Regional lymph node involvement (N)**
- NX: Regional lymph nodes cannot be assessed
- N0: No regional lymph node metastasis
- N1: Metastasis in a single regional lymph node[a]
- N2: Metastasis in more than one regional lymph node

**Distant metastasis (M)**
- MX: Distant metastasis cannot be assessed
- M0: No distant metastasis
- M1: Distant metastasis

[a] Laterality does not affect the N classification.

---

lymphatically. Box 8.1 and Table 8.1 give tumor–node–metastasis (TNM) definitions and stage groups for RCC.

**Treatment**   The mainstay of treatment for kidney cancer is surgery. Early stage disease is often treated with radical nephrectomy which will include removal of the kidney, adrenal gland, perirenal fat, and Gerota's fascia, with or without a regional lymph node dissection. For selected patients with a small tumor confined to the kidney, partial nephrectomy may be an option. External beam radiotherapy can be used, both pre- and postoperatively, but is often only palliative. Patients with later stage disease may benefit from embolization of the tumor, but again this is generally seen as a palliative measure. Response to cytotoxic chemotherapy is generally poor, but progress has been made with the intervention of biological therapies. Interferon alfa and interleukin-2 seem to be the two most effective of these therapies. Renal cell cancer is one

**Table 8.1** RCC—stage groups

| Stage | Primary tumor | Regional node involvement | Distant metastasis |
|-------|---------------|---------------------------|--------------------|
| I | T1 | N0 | M0 |
| II | T2 | N0 | M0 |
| III | T1 | N1 | M0 |
| | T2 | N1 | M0 |
| | T3 | N0 | M0 |
| | T3 | N1 | M0 |
| | T3a | N0 | M0 |
| | T3a | N1 | M0 |
| | T3b | N0 | M0 |
| | T3b | N1 | M0 |
| | T3c | N0 | M0 |
| | T3c | N1 | M0 |
| IV | T4 | N0 | M0 |
| | T4 | N1 | M0 |
| | Any T | N2 | M0 |
| | Any T | Any N | M1 |

of the few tumors in which spontaneous tumor regression in the absence of therapy exists, although these instances are rare.

Prognosis is directly related to the stage or degree of tumor dissemination. RCC confined to the kidney and surrounding area is often curable. Although some patients with regional lymphatic involvement achieve prolonged survival, involvement of lymphatic groups and the presence of distant metastases are associated with poor prognosis. Generally, patients present early while the disease is still localized, and therefore overall survival at 5 years is approximately 40%.

### Renal pelvis tumors

Because of the anatomical relationship between the renal pelvis and ureter, it is useful to consider these two sites together. Histologically, the two share the same basic type of epithelial lining, namely transitional cell epithelium or urothelium. The majority of renal pelvis and ureteric tumors are transitional cell carcinomas, with the occasional squamous cell carcinoma presenting. These tumors account for only a small percentage of kidney tumors and tend to be curable if diagnosed early enough. Some of the tumors that present are multifocal in origin, and the treatment is therefore designed to take this into account. Where multifocal disease of the renal pelvis and ureters is present, the probability of bladder involvement increases significantly.

**Staging**   The staging of these tumors is very similar to that of bladder cancer (see later) in that the important characteristic is the depth of invasion of the tumor in the renal pelvis or ureter (Box 8.2 and Table 8.2).

---

**Box 8.2**   Staging of renal pelvis and ureter tumors—TNM definitions

**Primary tumor (T)**
- TX: Primary tumor cannot be assessed
- T0: No evidence of primary tumor
- Ta: Papillary non-invasive carcinoma
- Tis: Carcinoma in situ
- T1: Tumor invades subepithelial connective tissue
- T2: Tumor invades the muscularis
- T3 (for renal pelvis only): Tumor invades beyond muscularis into peripelvic fat or the renal parenchyma
- T3 (for ureter only): Tumor invades beyond muscularis into periureteric fat
- T4: Tumor invades adjacent organs or through the kidney into perinephric fat

**Regional lymph node involvement (N)**
- NX: Regional lymph nodes cannot be assessed
- N0: No regional lymph node metastasis
- N1: Metastasis in a single lymph node, 2 cm or less in greatest dimension[a]
- N2: Metastasis in a single lymph node, more than 2 cm but not more than 5 cm in greatest dimension; or multiple lymph nodes, none more than 5 cm in greatest dimension
- N3: Metastasis in a lymph node, more than 5 cm in greatest dimension

**Distant metastasis (M)**
- MX: Distant metastasis cannot be assessed
- M0: No distant metastasis
- M1: Distant metastasis

[a] Laterality does not affect the N classification.

---

**Table 8.2**   Renal pelvis and ureter tumors—stage groups

| Stage | Primary tumor | Regional node involvement | Distant metastasis |
|-------|---------------|---------------------------|--------------------|
| 0a    | Ta            | N0                        | M0                 |
| 0is   | Tis           | N0                        | M0                 |
| I     | T1            | N0                        | M0                 |
| II    | T2            | N0                        | M0                 |
| III   | T3            | N0                        | M0                 |
| IV    | T4            | N0                        | M0                 |
|       | Any T         | N1                        | M0                 |
|       | Any T         | N2                        | M0                 |
|       | Any T         | N3                        | M0                 |
|       | Any T         | Any N                     | M1                 |

**Treatment**  Treatment for these tumors consists primarily of surgery. Generally, unless highly localized disease can be proved, total nephroureterectomy with removal of the bladder cuff is necessary. In selected patients partial removal can be undertaken.

Patients presenting with superficial tumors have a high percentage chance of cure (approximately 90%). Of those patients with more deeply invasive disease there is a 10–15% likelihood of cure; however, if the ureteric wall has been breached and/or there are metastases present, the likelihood of cure is very poor.

## Wilms' tumor (nephroblastoma)

Wilms' tumor is a malignant tumor of the kidney which affects children, typically between the ages of 1 and 5 years. Through the development of effective chemotherapy regimens and the advent of a multidisciplinary approach to these patients, the cure rates have significantly improved. Wilms' tumors seem to result from embryonic kidney tissue which has been retained, and this retained tissue has been associated with genetic defects, particularly located on the short arm of chromosome 11. Histological varieties such as anaplastic tumor, rhabdoid sarcoma, and clear cell sarcoma tend to have a worse prognosis than other histologies, such as multicystic nephroblastoma.

**Staging**  The staging system is based on the clinical findings determined by the pediatric surgeon at the time of operation. Histological features are also an important determinant of treatment and overall prognosis; well and moderately differentiated tumors are considered as 'favorable' histologies and anaplastic and sarcomatous as 'unfavorable'. Table 8.3 shows staging criteria for Wilms' tumor.

**Table 8.3**  Staging of Wilms' tumor

| Stage | Clinical findings |
| --- | --- |
| I | Tumor limited to the kidney and completely excised. Renal capsule is intact. The tumor is not ruptured before or during removal |
| II | Tumor extends beyond the kidney but is completely excised. No residual tumor is apparent at or beyond the margins of excision |
| III | Residual tumor confined to the abdomen—for example, peritoneal contamination or lymph node involvement |
| IV | Presence of hematogenous metastases, e.g. to the lung, liver, bone, or brain, or to a combination of these sites |
| V | Bilateral renal involvement at the time of initial diagnosis |

**Treatment**    Successful treatment of children with Wilms' tumor is very much dependent on the operations of the multidisciplinary team. Pediatric surgeon, radiation oncologist, radiographer, nurses, rehabilitation specialist, and others, working together in an effective team give the best chance of long-term cure for these patients. Because of the rarity of this disease patients should be treated in specialist centers.

Treatment consists of surgery, chemotherapy, and radiotherapy, alone or in combination. Surgery involves total nephrectomy. It is important that the surgeon does not rupture the kidney on removal as this may cause spread with the consequence of poorer prognosis. Where residual disease is left, it is generally marked with clips to aid in planning for radiotherapy treatment. For early stage disease, external beam radiotherapy is contraindicated, with adequate doses of vincristine and dactinomycin providing a good chance of long-term survival. It has been shown that stage III disease benefits from the addition of doxorubicin to the chemotherapy regimen, and low dose radiation therapy to the abdomen may be considered. Preoperative chemotherapy may be used for late and extensive disease in order to reduce the operable size of the tumor; however, this does have implications for the clinical staging of the disease at operation. Very young children (<12 months) should receive lower doses of chemotherapy drugs.

The prognosis for patients with Wilms' tumor is related not only to the specific features of the tumor and patient's age, but also to the workings of the multidisciplinary team as outlined earlier. Ninety percent of patients with favorable histology survive for 4 years. The cure rate for unfavorable histologies has also improved significantly with the addition of doxorubicin to the chemotherapy regimen.

## THE URINARY BLADDER

The urinary bladder is a reservoir for urine. It is a hollow muscular organ situated behind the symphysis pubis. In the male, the bladder is separated from the rectum (which lies behind) by the rectovesical fascia (Denonvillier's fascia), which contains the seminal vesicles and vas deferens. Below the bladder is the prostate gland, which encloses the first part of the urethra. In the female, the bladder lies in front of the vagina and the uterus, which also extends over the top of the bladder. The uterus and bladder are separated

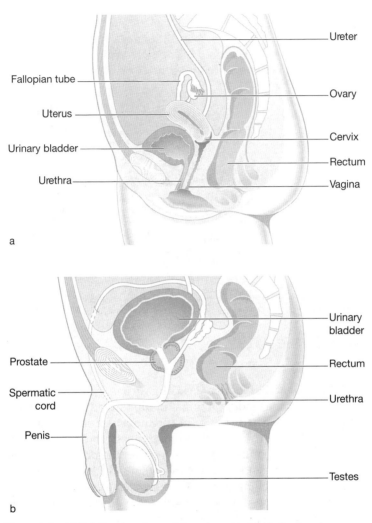

**Figure 8.3** (a) Relational anatomy of the urinary bladder in the female. (b) Relational anatomy of the urinary bladder in the male.

by a fold of peritoneum called the uterovesical pouch. The relational anatomy is shown in more detail in Figures 8.3a and 8.3b.

The bladder consists of an inner mucosa, typically transitional cell epithelium, or urothelium, which is generally in folds known as rugae. A triangular area known as the trigone is easily identifiable by the two ureters which enter the bladder, and the urethra

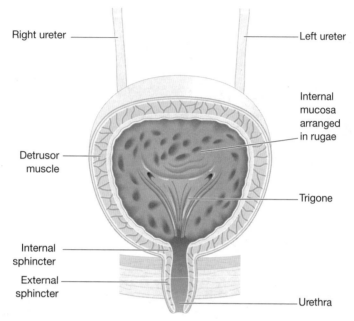

**Figure 8.4**  The urinary bladder.

which leaves it at the bladder neck. This area is typically smoother than the rest of the bladder lining and dips slightly in the ureter–urethra direction. The majority of carcinomas of the bladder are found in this area. The submucosa helps attach the mucosa to the thick muscle layer of the bladder known as the detrusor muscle. This is made up of smooth (involuntary) muscle that contracts the bladder when expelling urine. A final, outer layer, which covers only the superior portion of the bladder is sometimes referred to as the serosa or adventitia (see Fig. 8.4).

## Oncology

Carcinoma of the bladder accounts for 3–4% of all malignancies. The male to female ratio is approximately 4:1, and the disease usually occurs between the ages of 55 and 80 years. Although generally unknown, the cause may be linked to certain factors. The increase in environmental carcinogens and, in particular, 2-naphthylamine in the production of aniline dyes is a known risk factor. Workers in these industries have regular cytological screening for early

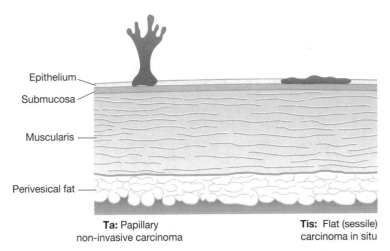

Ta: Papillary
non-invasive carcinoma

Tis: Flat (sessile)
carcinoma in situ

**Figure 8.5** Superficial and invasive tumors of the bladder. (After Fritz A. *Workbook for cancer staging.* 2nd edn. Lenexa, Kansas: National Cancer Registrars Association; 1999.)

detection. Smokers are also six times more likely to develop bladder cancer. The majority of cancers of the bladder are transitional cell (urothelial) carcinomas, with some adenocarcinomas and lymphomas occurring. Squamous cell carcinoma is rare in the UK, but can occur as a result of exposure to schistosomes, parasitic worms common in Egypt and central Africa.

Macroscopically, the disease can be divided into superficial (often referred to as papillary) carcinoma and solid carcinoma, which tends to be nodular in appearance and more infiltrative. *Papillary tumors* have narrow stalks and project into the lumen of the bladder. If they are confined to the surface of the epithelium they are described as non-invasive, but once the submucosa is involved, the tumor is frankly invasive. Solid or *sessile tumors* appear as flat lesions confined to the mucosal lining of the bladder and are described as carcinomas in situ (see Fig. 8.5).

### Staging

As previously described, the staging of bladder cancer is strongly related to the depth of invasion of the tumor (Box 8.3, Table 8.4 and Fig. 8.6) and has a marked effect on the management of the disease. Often tumors present with multifocal origin, and this has to be taken into account in deciding on the treatment regimen.

---

**Box 8.3** Staging of carcinoma of the bladder—TNM definitions

**Primary tumor (T)**
- TX: Primary tumor cannot be assessed
- T0: No evidence of primary tumor
- Ta: Papillary non-invasive carcinoma
- Tis: Carcinoma in situ: 'flat tumor'
- T1: Tumor invades subepithelial connective tissue
- T2: Tumor invades the muscularis—superficial (inner half) or deep (outer half)
  - —T2a: Tumor invades superficial muscle (inner half)
  - —T2b: Tumor invades deep muscle (outer half)
- T3: Tumor invades beyond perivesical tissue
  - —T3a: microscopically
  - —T3b: macroscopically (extravesical mass)
- T4: Tumor invades adjacent organs (prostate, uterus, vagina, pelvic wall, abdominal wall)
  - —T4a: Tumor invades prostate, uterus, vagina
  - —T4b: Tumor invades pelvic wall, abdominal wall

**Regional lymph node involvement (N)**
- NX: Regional lymph nodes cannot be assessed
- N0: No regional lymph node metastasis
- N1: Metastasis in a single lymph node, 2 cm or less in greatest dimension[a]
- N2: Metastasis in a single lymph node, more than 2 cm but not more than 5 cm in greatest dimension; or multiple lymph nodes, none more than 5 cm in greatest dimension
- N3: Metastasis in a lymph node more than 5 cm in greatest dimension

**Distant metastasis (M)**
- MX: Distant metastasis cannot be assessed
- M0: No distant metastasis
- M1: Distant metastasis

[a] Laterality does not affect the N classification.

---

**Table 8.4** Bladder carcinoma—stage groups

| Stage | Primary tumor | Regional node involvement | Distant metastasis |
|-------|---------------|---------------------------|--------------------|
| 0a    | Ta            | N0                        | M0                 |
| 0is   | Tis           | N0                        | M0                 |
| I     | T1            | N0                        | M0                 |
| II    | T2a           | N0                        | M0                 |
|       | T2b           | N0                        | M0                 |
| III   | T3a           | N0                        | M0                 |
|       | T3b           | N0                        | M0                 |
|       | T4a           | N0                        | M0                 |
| IV    | T4b           | N0                        | M0                 |
|       | Any T         | N1                        | M0                 |
|       | Any T         | N2                        | M0                 |
|       | Any T         | N3                        | M0                 |
|       | Any T         | Any N                     | M1                 |

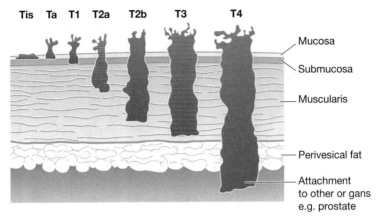

**Figure 8.6**   Staging of bladder cancer is based on depth of invasion through the bladder wall.

## Treatment

Treatment for carcinoma of the bladder is strongly related to the stage of the disease and consists of surgery, radiotherapy, and chemotherapy, in combination or alone.

*Superficial tumors* (Ta/T1) are removed by transurethral resection (TUR) or diathermy (fulguration). External beam radiotherapy is rarely used in these cases, because of the high chance of recurrence. Regular cystoscopy follow-up with or without TUR/diathermy can be very successful. For recurrence or multifocal disease, chemotherapy with mitomycin C is effective, or immunotherapy with BCG (bacillus Calmette–Guérin) can be used as an alternative. These drugs tend to be given intravesically—that is, they are introduced into the bladder lumen via a urethral catheter.

For *invasive tumors* (T2–T4), surgery and radiotherapy are the standard treatments. T2 tumors may first be resected surgically by TUR, but this may be followed by radiotherapy if there is residual disease. Patients with poorly differentiated T2 tumors are likely to receive radiotherapy as the primary treatment. T3 tumors tend to invade too deeply to be treated by TUR. External beam radiotherapy is the treatment of choice, with salvage surgery as an option if required. T4 tumors tend to be treated with palliative radiotherapy. The exception may be T4a tumors, as they invade only locally to the vagina or prostate and can be treated as radically as a T3 tumor.

Adenocarcinomas and squamous cell carcinomas of the bladder tend to be insensitive to radiotherapy, and therefore the treatment of choice is surgery.

Prognosis is related to the depth of invasion of the tumor. Patients with superficial tumors can survive many years with regular follow-up.

## SELF-ASSESSMENT QUESTIONS

Answer true or false to the following. Answers are on page 244.

1. Adults normally excrete 1–1.5 liters of urine per day.
2. The kidneys are divided into an outer medulla and inner cortex.
3. Epithelial cells line the tubules of the nephron.
4. Neuroblastoma is a common cancer of the kidney.
5. Renal cell carcinoma is also referred to as hypernephroma.
6. Renal cell carcinoma predominantly arises in the proximal convoluted tubule of the kidney.
7. A renal cell carcinoma greater than 7 cm suggests a T1 tumor.
8. External beam radiotherapy plays a major role in the radical treatment of renal cell carcinoma.
9. Renal pelvic tumors are mainly transitional cell carcinomas.
10. The renal pelvis has the same epithelial lining as the ureter.
11. Staging of renal pelvis and ureteric tumors is based on the size of the tumor.
12. Total nephroureterectomy and removal of the bladder cuff is the mainstay of treatment for renal pelvis and ureteric tumors.
13. Wilms' tumor is a malignant tumor which mainly affects adults.
14. A Wilms' tumor confined to the kidney and completely excised is indicative of a late stage tumor.
15. Few patients survive a Wilms' tumor.
16. The urinary bladder produces urine.
17. The urinary bladder is lined with transitional cell epithelium.
18. The majority of tumors of the bladder arise in the trigone area.
19. Squamous cell carcinoma is the most common malignancy of the bladder.
20. Treatment of carcinoma of the bladder is related to the depth of invasion of the tumor through the bladder wall.

# 9

# The male reproductive system

Anatomically, the main distinction between the male and female reproductive systems is the presence of visible male external genitalia, whereas in the female the reproductive organs lie within the pelvic cavity. The male reproductive system (Fig. 9.1) is composed of organs that are concerned with the production, maturation, and transfer of mature sperm into the female reproductive system to achieve fertilization. Production is initiated in the testes, and the resulting sperm are transferred from the testes via a duct system where the sperm gradually mature and are stored until they are expelled through the dual-functioning penis, which also transfers urine from the urinary bladder. Accessory reproductive glands produce most of the fluid, or semen, that transports and nourishes the sperm. These include the seminal vesicles, bulbourethral glands (Cowper's glands), and the prostate.

## THE TESTES

The testes (see Fig. 9.2) are a pair of small oval organs, about 5 cm in length and weighing 10–15 grams. They develop high on the posterior wall of the abdomen at the level of the kidney. Toward the end the 7th month of fetal development the testes usually descend into the pelvic cavity, through the peritoneum, and through a small inguinal opening or canal, out of the body and into the scrotum. As the testes pass through the abdomen they bring with them their own connective tissue composed of a cremaster muscle, blood, lymph, and nerve supply, and the vas deferens; these structures are known collectively as the spermatic cord and

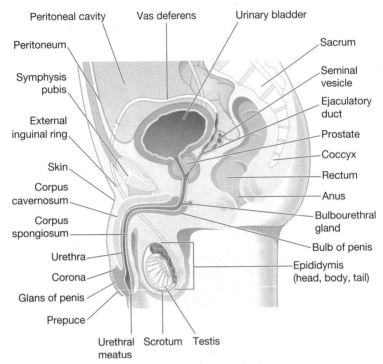

**Figure 9.1**   Relational anatomy of the male reproductive system.

hold the testes suspended in the scrotal sac. As the testes pass through the inguinal canal they acquire peritoneal coverings: a thin outer serous layer called the tunica vaginalis (which also lines the inner scrotal sacs) and a thicker fibrous, white, inner layer called the tunica albuginea that also extends into the mass of the testicular tissue and divides it into 200–300 compartments called lobules (see Fig. 9.2). Each of these lobules contains:

- specialized interstitial cells called Leydig cells (which secrete male hormones or androgens, especially testosterone) and Sertoli cells that regulate metabolism and provide support and nourishment of the developing sperm
- seminiferous tubules—within each lobule are between one and four small coiled seminiferous tubules where sperm production is initiated (spermatogenesis).

The tubules from each lobule join together to form a plexus of vessels called the rete (pronounced ree-tee) testis; these drain into a series of sperm ducts called the efferent ducts, which pierce the

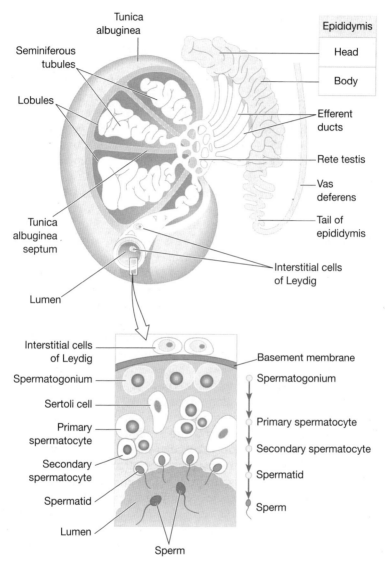

**Figure 9.2** Anatomy of the testis and scrotum.

tunica vaginalis and converge to become the head of the epididymis. The *epididymis* is a tightly coiled tube encased in a fibrous layer; it is comma-shaped and lies superior and posterior to the testis. The epididymis is composed of a head, body, and tail that are continuous with the vas deferens. The epididymis acts as a duct through which sperm pass, but it also stores the sperm for 1–3 weeks while they mature, and it secretes a small part of the seminal fluid (semen). The developing young sperm or spermatozoa require a cooler temperature than the rest of the body, and two muscles assist this process: the smooth dartos muscle from the scrotum, which causes the scrotal skin to wrinkle; and the cremaster muscle, which lies in the spermatic cord and allows the testes to rise or fall to maintain the temperature at 3°C below core body temperature.

The descent of the testes into the scrotum is critically important for sperm production; failure of this to happen is known as cryptorchidism (hidden testes, or maldescent). *Cryptorchidism* occurs in about 3% of full-term babies and about 30% of premature babies and may be unilateral (one-sided) or bilateral (involving both testes). If bilateral cryptorchidism is left untreated, sterility will result, because the body's core temperature is 3°C higher than in the scrotal sac. However, about 80% of maldescended testes will spontaneously descend during the first year of life. If this does not occur, surgical intervention (orchidopexy) is necessary before the male infant reaches 18 months. A history of cryptorchidism is a strong risk factor for developing testicular cancer. Because the testes originate high on the upper abdominal wall, the lymphatic drainage differs from that of the surrounding scrotum. This is very important, as the routes of spread and treatment management reflect this difference. Thus the testis, because of its original embryonic site of origin in the abdomen, initially drains along the spermatic cord, then up to the para-aortic nodes, into the retroperitoneal and retrocrural nodes, then through the diaphragm and into the thoracic duct via the posterior mediastinum and supraclavicular nodes (usually left-sided), and eventually back into the main blood system.

The scrotal sac, however, drains first to regional nodes, then into inguinal nodes, so a surgical procedure to access the testes through the scrotal sac (trans-scrotal orchidectomy) is not advised. The preferred access is through a high incision in the inguinal area to prevent the risk of scrotal recurrence or later inguinal node involvement.

## Oncology

Testicular cancer is the most common solid tumor among young men aged 15–39 years. In 2001, an estimated 7200 new cases of testicular cancer were diagnosed in the USA and about 1500 in the

UK, with an estimated 400 deaths in the USA. The three age ranges associated with testicular cancer are: a small peak in childhood (0–10 years), a major peak at 15–39 years, and a smaller peak at around 60 years. The survival rate has risen from 79% in the 1970s to more than 95% in the 1990s because of improved treatment regimens.

## Histology

Testicular tumors tend to be rapidly growing and can have a doubling time of 20–30 days. The great majority of testicular tumors, 90–95%, are germ cell tumors (GCTs). These GCTs are classified into two groups: seminomas and non-seminomas, along with mixed cell tumors (Box 9.1). The remaining testicular tumors (5–10%) consist of lymphomas and other tumors arising from the Leydig and Sertoli cells. GCTs often contain malignant cells and tissue that closely resembles normal embryological tissue. GCTs are often able to secrete specialized hormones, such as alfa-fetoprotein (AFP) and human chorionic gonadotropin (HCG), that are normally produced by germ cells in the developing fetus (see Ch. 1). AFP and HCG can be used as tumor markers, as they are useful in monitoring how well the patient's tumor responds to any therapy.

*Seminomas* arise from cells that support spermatogenesis (generation of sperm) in the seminiferous tubules, and they are the most common form of testicular cancer. Seminomas are divided into three groups:

• Classic seminoma is most common in men in their 30s and is associated with increased secretion of HCG. A pure seminoma does not secrete AFP.

• Anaplastic seminoma is similar to the classic type but is often more advanced. About 30% of testicular cancer deaths occur from

---

**Box 9.1**    North American classification and distribution of testicular cancers

| Seminoma (35%) | Non-seminoma (40%) | Other (~25%) |
|---|---|---|
| • Classic (most common) | • Embryonal cell carcinoma (most common) | • Mixed cell tumors—elements of both seminomas and non-seminomas |
| • Anaplastic | • Teratoma | • Lymphomas |
| • Spermatocytic | • Choriocarcinoma | • Leydig cell and Sertoli cell tumors |
| | • Yolk sac tumor (endodermal sinus) | |

this type, due to the increased microinvasion and greater cellular anaplasia of the tumor. About 46% present with extragonadal disease, and HCG levels are higher than for classic seminoma.

• Spermatocytic seminoma is a rare type found in men in their 50s. It is thought to arise from the developing sperm and is treated by orchidectomy, which is usually curative.

*Non-seminomas* tend to be more common in younger men (in their 20s) and constitute approximately 40% of all testicular cancers. In 90% of non-seminomas, a tumor marker is secreted which is very useful in monitoring therapy. There are four classifications of non-seminomas:

• Embryonal carcinoma. Often these tumors are very small, even when advanced. They can contain embryonal tissue resembling a 1–2-week-old embryo and also have trophoblastic or yolk sac elements. Embryonal carcinoma can produce increased secretion of AFP, HCG, or both. These tumors tend to be quite aggressive and have a high potential for metastasis.

• Teratomas are technically non-malignant but can metastasize. They do not secrete AFP or HCG but may show differentiation toward all three embryological germ cell layers—the ectoderm, mesoderm, and endoderm—although this is usually less marked than in ovarian teratoma, which often differentiates into fully mature tissue.

• Choriocarcinoma is the most aggressive type of germ cell tumor in adults, producing widespread metastases and lymphatic spread, with normal AFP levels but elevated HCG.

• Yolk sac tumors account for the majority of testicular tumors found in children under 15 years. In its purest form, a yolk sac tumor is highly likely to metastasize to the liver. Yolk sac tumors produce normal HCG and raised levels of AFP, which can be used to monitor response to treatment and the status of disease.

Tumors consisting of two or more cell types make up the rest. The characteristics of various types of testicular tumors are summarized in Table 9.1.

### Etiology

**Cryptorchidism** A history of cryptorchidism is the most important risk factor and is present in 10% of all testicular cancers. Maldescent may be part of an initiating event that leads to

**Table 9.1** Characteristics of different types of testicular tumors

|  | Seminoma | Embryonal | Teratoma | Choriocarcinoma |
|---|---|---|---|---|
| Potential for metastasis | Low | Medium | Low; late relapse | High |
| Route of spread | Lymphatic | Blood/lymph | Lymphatic | Blood |
| Rate of doubling | Months | Weeks | Months | 24 hours |
| AFP secretion | − | +/− | − | − |
| HCG secretion | +/− | +/− | − | +++ |
| LDH secretion | +/− | +/− | +/− | +/− |
| Chemosensitivity | + | + | Less | + |
| Radiosensitivity | +++ | Less | Less | Less |

AFP, alfa-fetoprotein; HCG, human chorionic gonadotropin; LDH, lactate dehydrogenase.

testicular cancer. There is a 15–20% increase in the risk of developing carcinoma in situ in the contralateral testicle. The location where the developing testicle lodges in the abdomen can affect the risk of developing cancer, as an abdominal cryptorchid testicle (where the maldescended testis may be stuck inside the abdominal cavity) is four times more likely to develop cancer than an inguinal testicle. There is also an association with testicular torsion and inguinal hernias. Seventy percent of bilateral cryptorchidisms will result in sterility. An operation called orchiopexy (surgically descending the testicle) does not reduce the risk of cancer but allows for examination and earlier detection.

**Carcinoma in situ**   This is a precursor to most GCTs and may be referred to as intratubular germ cell neoplasia. Carcinoma in situ may occur during fetal development; proliferation and invasion occur after puberty and may well be hormone-induced.

**History of a previous testicular cancer**   There is a 5% risk of contralateral involvement, and carcinoma in situ may be present contralaterally in 10% of patients. If the patient had bilateral cryptorchidism with a previous history of testicular cancer, there is a 25% chance of contralateral involvement.

**Atrophic testis**   Atrophy of the testis (dysgenesis) carries an increased risk of cancer and can be due to congenital causes, feminization syndromes, viral causes, or testicular atrophy. Feminization syndrome results from an overproduction of female hormones or underproduction of male hormones, causing development of female characteristics, such as breast enlargement (gynecomastia).

For example, Klinefelter's syndrome is closely associated with mediastinal GCTs. The increase in the risk of developing testicular cancer is 40-fold in patients who demonstrate testicular feminization syndromes. Viral causes include human immunodeficiency virus (HIV). Testicular atrophy following an infection of mumps is identified as giving a small increased risk of developing cancer.

**Primary relatives with testicular cancer history**   In up to one third of cases, a genetic link is implicated. This is supported by the protective effect of African-American lineage and by a chromosomal deletion on chromosome 12 found in many patients with seminoma, non-seminoma, and carcinoma in situ. Also, a recently located gene, *TGCT1*, makes men who carry it more susceptible to testicular germ cell cancers (TGCT), which constitute 95% of all testicular cancer cases.

As the testes descend from the posterior wall of the abdomen, they take their blood and lymphatic drainage from the area of origin, so that any involvement of the lymphatic system will spread directly to the para-aortic lymph node chain that lies alongside the vertebral column at the level of the kidneys. Involvement of nodes such as the internal and external iliac nodes suggests that there may be local extension from the tumor involving other structures. TNM definitions and stage groups are given in Boxes 9.2a and 9.2b, and Table 9.2.

## Clinical features

The usual initial finding is heaviness or a painless lump in or on the testis, or a change in texture of the testicular tissue, such as hardness, or the testis may become enlarged. Less commonly, there is associated pain and tenderness. Other symptoms, such as hemoptysis, back pain, and loin pain or neck lymphadenopathy unfortunately suggest widespread metastatic disease, and about 10% of patients may present with one or more of these symptoms. A relatively large proportion of patients having occult metastatic disease may not display any of these sinister symptoms at the time of diagnosis. AFP and HCG levels in the blood can be raised, indicating the presence of an active germ cell tumor. Most testicular cancer is diagnosed through self-examination, a process whereby the male regularly examines the testes for any signs of abnormality. Testicular self-examination is best attended to directly after a hot bath or shower when the muscles are at their

---

**Box 9.2a**   Staging of testicular tumors—TNM definitions[a]

**Primary tumor (T)**
- pTX: Primary tumor cannot be assessed (if no radical orchidectomy has been performed, TX is used)
- pT0: No evidence of primary tumor (e.g. histological scar in testis)
- pTis: Intratubular germ cell neoplasia (carcinoma in situ)
- pT1: Tumor limited to testis and epididymis without lymphatic/vascular invasion
- pT2: Tumor limited to testis with epididymis with lymphatic/vascular invasion, or tumor extending through the tunica albuginea with involvement of tunica vaginalis
- pT3: Tumor invades the spermatic cord with or without vascular/lymphatic invasion
- pT4: Tumor invades the scrotum with/without vascular/lymphatic invasion

**Regional lymph node involvement (N)**
- cNX: Regional lymph nodes cannot be assessed
- cN0: No regional lymph node metastasis
- cN1: Metastasis in a single lymph node, 2 cm or less in greatest dimension, or multiple lymph nodes, none more than 2 cm in greatest dimension
- cN2: Metastasis with a lymph node mass more than 2 cm but not more than 5 cm in greatest dimension; or multiple lymph nodes, any one mass greater than 2 cm but not more than 5 cm in greatest dimension
- cN3: Metastasis in a lymph node mass more than 5 cm in greatest dimension

**Distant metastasis (M)**
- MX: Presence of distant metastasis cannot be assessed
- M0: No distant metastasis
- M1: Distant metastasis
  —M1a: Non-regional nodal or pulmonary metastasis
  —M1b: Distant metastasis other than to non-regional nodes and lungs

[a]The stage grouping for testicular cancer requires additional information about serum markers (S)—see Box 9.2b.

---

**Box 9.2b**   Serum tumor markers (S)

- SX: Marker studies not available or not performed
- S0: Marker study levels within normal range
- S1: LDH $< 1.5 \times$ N $and$ HCG $< 5000$ mIu/ml $and$ AFP $< 1000$ ng/ml
- S2: LDH $1.5–10 \times$ N $or$ HCG $5–50 \times 10^3$ mIu/ml $or$ AFP $1–10 \times 10^3$ ng/ml
- S3: LDH $> 10 \times$ N $or$ HCG $> 50 \times 10^3$ mIu/ml $or$ AFP $> 10 \times 10^3$ ng/ml

AFP, alfa-fetoprotein; HCG, human chorionic gonadotropin; LDH, lactate dehydrogenase. N indicates the upper limit of normal for the LDH assay.

---

most relaxed. This allows the individual to become familiar with the normal texture of the testes and therefore any changes can be detected at a very early stage. This form of testicular screening is cheap, non-invasive, and easily reproducible; however, educating

**Table 9.2** Testicular cancer—stage groups

| Stage | Primary tumor | Regional node involvement | Distant metastasis | Serum tumor markers |
|---|---|---|---|---|
| 0 | pTis | N0 | M0 | S0 |
| I | pT1–4 | N0 | M0 | SX |
| IA | pT1 | N0 | M0 | S0 |
| IB | pT2 | N0 | M0 | S0 |
| | pT3 | N0 | M0 | S0 |
| | pT4 | N0 | M0 | S0 |
| IS | Any pT/TX | N0 | M0 | S1–3 |
| II | Any pT/TX | N1–3 | M0 | SX |
| IIA | Any pT/TX | N1 | M0 | S0 |
| | Any pT/TX | N1 | M0 | S1 |
| IIB | Any pT/TX | N2 | M0 | S0 |
| | Any pT/TX | N2 | M0 | S1 |
| IIC | Any pT/TX | N3 | M0 | S0 |
| | Any pT/TX | N3 | M0 | S1 |
| III | Any pT/TX | Any N | M1 | SX |
| IIIA | Any pT/TX | Any N | M1a | S0 |
| | Any pT/TX | Any N | M1a | S1 |
| IIIB | Any pT/TX | N1–3 | M0 | S2 |
| | Any pT/TX | Any N | M1a | S2 |
| IIIC | Any pT/TX | N1–3 | M0 | S3 |
| | Any pT/TX | Any N | M1a | S3 |
| | Any pT/TX | Any N | M1b | Any S |

young men to do this is a problem, so unfortunately not enough young males are doing self-examination. Consequently, late stages of this highly treatable and curative disease are still being found.

If cancer is suspected, biochemical tests for tumor markers can show very high levels of AFP and HCG; preoperative and post-operative measurements are helpful not only in diagnosis but in staging and monitoring the response of the tumor to treatment. Serum placental alkaline phosphatase is often raised in seminoma, but is not diagnostic as it may be raised for other reasons, such as smoking. Although a clinician can palpate the testis and ultrasound is useful to determine if the patient has testicular cancer, it is only after an inguinal orchidectomy that the testis can be directly seen and biopsies taken if necessary. Therefore, diagnosis is only con-firmed on biopsy. Often a chest X-ray is done to exclude the possi-bility of lung metastases, and a computed tomography (CT) scan is done to try and assess any local spread and possible lymphatic involvement; these evaluations are essential for correctly staging the disease and deciding the appropriate treatment.

**Table 9.3** A summary of the international germ cell prognostic classification devised for metastatic testicular carcinomas

| Prognosis | Seminoma | Non-seminoma |
|---|---|---|
| Good | Any primary site without pulmonary visceral metastases *and* with normal AFP, any HCG, any LDH (90% of seminomas): 5-year PFS 82%; 5-year survival 86% | Testis/retroperitoneal primary without pulmonary visceral metastases and with good markers of AFP < 1000 ng/ml *and* HCG < 5000 mIu/ml *and* LDH < 1.5 × upper limit of normal (56% of non-seminomas): 5-year PFS 89%; 5-year survival 92% |
| Intermediate | Any primary site without pulmonary visceral metastases *and* normal AFP, any HCG, any LDH (10% of seminomas): 5-year PFS 67%; 5-year survival 72% | Testis/retroperitoneal primary without pulmonary visceral metastases and with intermediate markers of AFP 1–10 × 10³ ng/ml *or* HCG 5–50 × 10³ mIu/ml *or* LDH 1.5–10 × N (28% of non-seminomas): 5-year PFS 75%; 5-year survival 80% |
| Poor | No patients are classified as poor prognosis | Mediastinal primary *or* pulmonary visceral metastases *or* poor markers of AFP > 10 × 10³ ng/ml *or* HCG > 50 × 10³ mIu/ml *or* LDH > 10 × N (16% of non-seminomas): 5-year PFS 41%; 5-year survival 48% |

AFP, alfa-fetoprotein; HCG, human chorionic gonadotropin; LDH, lactate dehydrogenase; PFS, progression-free survival. N indicates the upper limit of normal for the LDH assay.

### Treatment of testicular cancer

Testicular cancer is extremely treatable and is often curable, particularly in young and middle-aged men. Management is based on whether the tumor is of seminoma or non-seminoma type and is related to the tumor's manner of spread, as seminomas spread via the lymphatics and non-seminomas spread via the blood. Seminomas are also much more sensitive to radiation and respond well to radiotherapy treatment, unlike non-seminomas (see Table 9.3). When all stages of seminoma are combined, the cure rate is over 90%; if treated at an early stage, the cure rate is almost 100%.

All treatments have a similar pattern, with a radical inguinal orchidectomy performed first.

- For very early stage testicular seminomas (stage I), a surgical radical inguinal orchidectomy is followed by radiotherapy (because of seminomas' sensitivity to radiation) to the most likely route of lymphatic spread, i.e. the para-aortic nodes. Stage I seminoma has a cure rate of more than 95%.

- For stage I non-seminomas, a radical inguinal orchidectomy is followed by monthly serum marker checks and chest X-rays for 1 year and every 2 months in the second year. If the serum markers rise after orchidectomy, chemotherapy and/or radiotherapy can be used as salvage therapy.

- For higher stages of seminomas, treatment is determined by whether the tumor is bulky or non-bulky, where bulky is defined as tumor greater than 5 cm on CT scan. If the tumor is small (termed non-bulky), radiotherapy alone may be sufficient to treat the para-aortic and pelvic nodes, with cure rates of over 90%. If the seminoma is larger (termed bulky), then chemotherapy is followed by radiotherapy.

Tumor types with mixed cell types tend to have a poorer prognosis, more extensive disease, and high blood serum markers. These patients should receive more intensive regimens with weekly administration of alternating drug combinations. For recurrent or resistant cases, high dose chemotherapy should be used.

## PROSTATE GLAND

The prostate is an accessory gland of the reproductive system and consists of both glandular and muscular tissue. The prostate lies immediately below the bladder, anterior to the rectum and posterior to the pubic ramis. It is about the size of a walnut and is fully mature by the time a man reaches 30; the size remains stable until about the age of 45 when it commonly begins to enlarge (a condition called benign hypertrophy). The prostate is traversed by the urethra, which is lined with transitional cells, and by ejaculatory ducts from the seminal vesicles that join the vas deferens just before entering the prostate. The prostate is an encapsulated, glandular organ with numerous partitions, divided into three zones: peripheral, transitional, and central (see Fig. 9.3). The cells that line the partitions secrete prostatic fluid; this forms the bulk of seminal fluid and is a milky fluid of pH 7.4. This is slightly alkaline, which

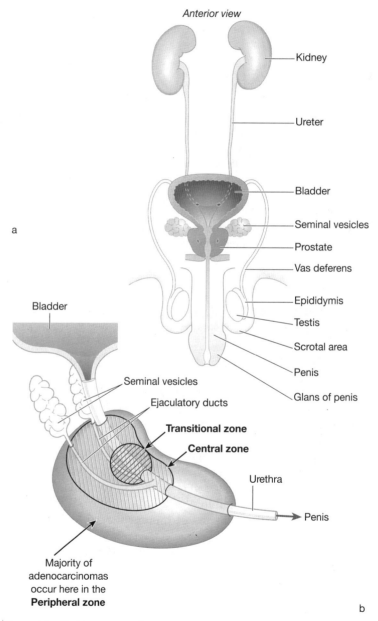

**Figure 9.3** The anatomy of the prostate gland: (a) relation to other organs (anterior view with non-uniform scale); (b) '3D' cross-section to show concentric zonal arrangement around the urethra: (i) central, (ii) transitional, (iii) peripheral.

is important as it protects the sperm from the acidic environment present in the male urethra and female vagina.

# Oncology

Cancer of the prostate is one of the most common cancers in males—about 30% of all new cancers diagnosed in males. The disease is rare before 40, and is probably related to the hyperplasia that occurs in the middle 40s. The most important factor in prostate cancer is its relatively high median age at diagnosis, with 70% of men diagnosed with prostatic cancer being over 65. About 1 in 6 men will be diagnosed with prostate cancer during his lifetime, but only 1 in 32 will die of it. Of men over 50 years, 30–40% have some form of prostate cancer, and 20–25% of these will progress to clinically detectable disease.

## Etiology

The underlying etiologic factors for prostate cancer are not known, but there are associated risk factors:

- androgens—in males castrated before puberty, prostate cancer is very rare
- genetic links, showing increasing risk with family history
- race-related factors—incidence is lower in Caucasians than in blacks. African-Americans have the highest incidence of prostate cancer in the world
- geographical variation between countries suggests genetic links are rare in Asia, Africa, South and Central America
- diet—higher incidence if diet is rich in fat, particularly red meat; low if rich in vitamin A
- environment—heavy metals, cadmium, nuclear industry, chemical fertilizers
- occult cancer—15% are discovered incidentally at prostatectomy for benign disease.

## Histology

The majority of prostate tumors are adenocarcinomas (95%). The peripheral zone (70–75% of the gland) is the largest zone of the prostate and accounts for 70% of prostate cancers. The transitional zone (5% of the gland) is the location where benign nodular hyperplasia develops, 20% of which may become adenocarcinoma. The central zone (20–25% of the gland) accounts for about 10% of prostate cancers. Rarely, transitional cell carcinoma arises in large ducts lined by transitional cells. Often the adenocarcinomas are well differentiated, though there can be variation throughout the organ. There can be a wide range of tumor differentiation and abnormal histological growth, and this is closely related to the likelihood of metastases and death. Because of this variability within the tumor, many pathologists report the range of differentiation present in the specimen using the Gleason grading scale that was developed over 20 years ago for the USA-based Veteran's Administration Cooperative Urological Research Group (VACURG).

### Clinical features

The symptoms of cancer are often indistinguishable from normal benign enlargement of the prostate. This is a common occurrence in men over the age of 50. The symptoms include increased difficulty in micturition (urination), loss of stream strength, hesitancy, post-micturition dribble, and the need to urinate frequently (frequency), especially at night (nocturia). About a third of patients present with local invasion and a range of symptoms that includes hematuria, tenesmus, impotence, incontinence, loin pain, anuria (inability to urinate), and lymphedema from acute urinary retention. About 7% of patients will present with metastatic spread, often with bone pain, pathological fracture, or sacral, sciatic, or perineal pain due to infiltration of nerves in the pelvis. Unfortunately, 75% of patients have some form of spread at presentation, half of them with distant metastases.

Direct spread of prostate cancer tends to be to adjacent organs: the bladder, seminal vesicles, and rectum. Lymphatic spread is via the obturator nodes located in the pelvis, then to presacral nodes that lie adjacent to the sacrum, then to internal and external iliac nodes, and then on to the para-aortics before joining the main collecting lymphatic trunk, called the cisterna chyli. Blood-borne spread is common as there is a rich venous plexus lying in front of the vertebral bodies, which may account for a tendency to spread to vertebrae and pelvic bones. Bone secondaries tend to be of a sclerotic type, which show as increased density on radiographs, as a result of new bone formation, and eventually invade lung tissue. A bone scan is an exceptionally useful investigative tool in showing up areas of increased density which may indicate increased metastatic activity (see later in the chapter).

### Screening

Prostatic cancer is variable in its behavior. In the more elderly patient, it may be a very indolent, well-differentiated tumor that is found incidentally at postmortem (30% of men over 50). It is often more aggressive in younger patients, especially if the tumor is poorly differentiated. Because of the frequency and clearly age-related development of prostate cancer, screening has been increasingly advocated.

Clinical examination by digital rectal examination (DRE) has a detection rate of 1%. However, the prostate secretes a special antigen specific only to the prostate that has been a very valuable tumor marker, as assays of prostate-specific antigen (PSA) correlate with the level and extent of disease. If a patient with localized disease is treated with a radical prostatectomy (removal of the prostate), the PSA level should fall below normal levels. Approximately 30% of men with a PSA level of 2–4 ng/ml will have prostate cancer confirmed on biopsy. Unfortunately, 20% of men with clinically significant prostate cancer will have normal levels of PSA. Although 60% of cancers that are detected have already spread beyond the prostate, screening with both PSA and DRE should be able to detect the tumor at an earlier stage when it is still confined to the gland. However, 14–35% of men with prostatic cancer will have normal levels of PSA, and 30% of men with cancer have normal DRE. Different authorities give different recommendations. The American Cancer Society recommends regular PSA level checks from the age of 50 years and regular DRE over 40 years, whereas medical authorities make no recommendations. So the problem remains whom to screen: should it be high risk populations? Those with a family history? Men over age 50, or 60, or 70, with more than 10 years of life expectancy? Even with screening, some cases may not be picked up, while other patients may suffer unnecessary side effects, or there may be a decision made not to treat after all. Consequently, the whole issue of screening is riddled with controversy.

*Diagnostic procedures*

- *DRE* can detect abnormalities—the gland feels irregular and hard. DRE is an inexpensive and non-morbid test, but it is limited and is more effective at detecting tumors in advanced stages. Between 20% and 25% of men with an abnormal DRE will have prostate cancer, but about 30% of men diagnosed with prostate cancer will have a normal DRE. So, following the DRE, a biopsy must be performed to confirm cancer, as benign hypertrophy can also cause the prostate to enlarge but feel smooth and firm.
- *PSA* is released by the prostate epithelium. It is an indicator of prostate activity, not of prostate cancer. However, PSA levels above 4 ng/ml indicate an increased probability of cancer. Certain non-cancerous conditions can also increase PSA levels, and there is a tendency for PSA levels to rise with age. PSA levels have to be adjusted for age, and they also vary with race. PSA testing should be done before any therapy is undertaken, because certain procedures can affect PSA levels—for example, a prostate biopsy can increase PSA. After treatment, PSA can be used as a marker to monitor the effectiveness of therapy.
- *Transrectal ultrasound* (TRUS) is not a screening tool but assists during the biopsy. A probe is inserted into the rectum and sound waves are used to identify small peripheral tumors and to guide the needle for biopsy core samples to be taken.

As so many patients are asymptomatic, it is important to assess the local extent of the disease as well as the possibility of distant metastases. An *isotope bone scan* is useful for identifying asymptomatic bone metastases, especially when occult metastases are present in the skull, ribs, or upper part of the spine. A bone scan is administered using an intravenous drip of a phosphorus-based compound attached to a radioactive agent labeled with technetium-99 m. The radioactive agent seeks out and is absorbed by bone after a period of 2–4 hours. Between 50% and 60% of the injection is deposited in the bony skeleton and the remainder is excreted by the kidneys. Where there is a lot of activity in bone, the bone scan will show these areas of increased uptake as dark 'hot spots'. If a patient has a negative bone scan but has increased levels of acid phosphatase, the incidence of pelvic nodal involvement is 60% higher than if the alkaline phosphatase is normal.

Prostate cancer staging uses the TNM system (see Box 9.3). However, grading (how well or poorly differentiated the tumor is)

---

**Box 9.3**   Staging of prostate cancer—TNM definitions

**Primary tumor (T)**
- TX: Primary tumor cannot be assessed
- T0: No evidence of primary tumor
- T1: Clinically inapparent tumor, not palpable and not visible by imaging
  —T1a: Tumor incidental histological finding in 5% or less of tissue resected at TURP
  —T1b: Tumor incidental histological finding in more than 5% of tissue resected at TURP
  —T1c: Tumor identified by needle biopsy (e.g. because of elevated PSA)
- T2 Tumor confined within prostate[a]
  —T2a: Tumor involves one half of one lobe or less
  —T2b: Tumor involves more than one half of one lobe but not both lobes
  —T2c: Tumor involves both lobes
- T3: Tumor extends through the prostatic capsule[b]
  —T3a: Extracapsular extension (unilateral or bilateral)
  —T3b: Tumor invades seminal vesicle(s)
- T4: Tumor is fixed or invades adjacent structures other than seminal vesicles: bladder neck, external sphincter, rectum, levator muscles, and/or pelvic wall

**Regional lymph node involvement (N)**
- NX: Regional lymph nodes cannot be assessed
- N0: No regional lymph node metastasis
- N1: Metastasis in regional lymph nodes

**Distant metastasis (M)**
- MX: Distant metastasis cannot be assessed
- M0: No distant metastasis
- M1: Distant metastasis
  —M1a: Non-regional lymph node(s)
  —M1b: Bone(s)
  —M1c: Other site(s) with or without bone disease

[a]Tumor found in one or both lobes by needle biopsy, but not palpable or reliably visible by imaging, is classified as T1c.
[b]Invasion into the prostatic apex or into (but not beyond) the prostatic capsule is classified not as T3 but as T2.

---

is important as an indicator of how slowly or quickly the disease may progress; in other words, it assesses the degree of aggressiveness of the tumor. The *Gleason scale* provides a measure of this. The higher the Gleason score, the more likelihood of extracapsular spread, nodal involvement, and metastatic disease. The Gleason score, based on the Gleason grade, provides prognostic information (see Table 9.4). The prostate tumor samples are reviewed under the microscope. A dominant pattern is identified and given a number between 1 and 5, then a secondary pattern is identified and given a number between 1 and 5. These pattern numbers are added together to give an overall score (between

**Table 9.4**   The Gleason grading scale for prostate cancer

| Gleason score | Differentiation | Chance of local progression by 10 years (%) | Chance of death from cancer by 15 years (%) |
|---|---|---|---|
| 2–4 | Good | 25 | 8 |
| 5–6 | Moderate | 50 | 35 |
| 7–10 | Poor | 70 | 65 |

2 and 10) that can predict disease progression and determine what is the most appropriate treatment. Well differentiated prostate cancers may have a very long, slow progression. Patient are often elderly (late 70–80s), and because the disease has a development period of more than 10 years before the patient shows any symptoms, he may well die of other causes. Higher Gleason scores often indicate a more active tumor that requires more intensive forms of treatment. Stage groups for prostatic cancer are given in Table 9.5.

## Treatment

To determine the most appropriate treatment, clinical tumor (T) stage, Gleason score and pre-treatment PSA level are combined and taken into account. Other factors that affect treatment decisions are the patient's age, personal preference, and health status. The aim of treatment is to control spread and reduce tumor cells, to allow the patient to live out his life untroubled by disease.

**Table 9.5**   Prostate cancer—stage groups

| Stage | Primary tumor | Regional node involvement | Distant metastasis | G[a] |
|---|---|---|---|---|
| I | T1a | N0 | M0 | G1 |
| II | T1a | N0 | M0 | G2, G3–4 |
| | T1b | N0 | M0 | Any G |
| | T1c | N0 | M0 | Any G |
| | T1 | N0 | M0 | Any G |
| | T2 | N0 | M0 | Any G |
| III | T3 | N0 | M0 | Any G |
| IV | T4 | N0 | M0 | Any G |
| | Any T | N1 | M0 | Any G |
| | Any T | Any N | M1 | Any G |

[a]G refers to the degree of differentiation, which can be gauged through the Gleason score (see Table 9.4): G1, Gleason score 2–4; G2, Gleason score 5–6; G3–4, Gleason score 7–10.

In men with localized prostate cancer and a life expectancy of at least 10 years, there are two main treatment options: radical prostatectomy or radiation therapy. The normal prostate will tolerate high doses of radiation without prostatic symptoms, making external beam radiotherapy a possible treatment option for localized disease. However, there are critical organs adjacent to the prostate that are very vulnerable to radiation damage and this can cause serious problems. Brachytherapy is commonly used as an alternative to external beam radiotherapy treatment. The use of implanted radioactive iodine-131 allows a high dose of radiation to be given to the prostate itself with minimal doses to surrounding normal structures. This technique has demonstrated fewer side effects than surgery and external beam radiotherapy, particularly with regard to sexual function. The prognosis for prostate cancer is particularly difficult to assess, because of the uncertain progress of the disease and the naturally high death rate in this group of elderly men. Cure is difficult to define in an elderly population; 5-year survival for T1–2 cases is about 78% and for T3, about 59%.

**Treatment options for localized and metastatic disease** The prostate, like the breast, is hormonally influenced. This was discovered by Huggins in 1941. Prostatic cancer can be treated with hormone therapy in a number of ways:

- removal of male hormones through orchidectomy
- administration of female hormones (estrogens)
- administration of chemicals that reduce testosterone production—luteinizing hormone-releasing hormone (LHRH), which diminishes pituitary production of gonadotropin and eventually leads to a drop in testosterone production
- blocking the action of androgens through oral agents.

Eighty percent of patients will respond to hormone therapy, and starting hormone therapy early seems to delay the onset of symptoms. Unfortunately, it does not improve overall survival, and 70% of patients with bone metastases will die within 2 years of diagnosis. Palliative radiotherapy is good at giving relief from bone pain and is useful for shrinking locally advanced disease to reduce symptoms of urinary obstruction, lymphedema and nerve compression. Radiotherapy can also be used to prevent gynecomastia in patients given diethylstilbestrol; this can also give patients a psychological boost. In hormone-resistant cases, radiotherapy also seems to have no effect, so alternative pain control and support are required.

## PENIS

The penis has two functions: depositing sperm in the female reproductive tract, and acting as the terminal duct for the urinary tract, to allow the elimination of urine. It consists of an attached root, a free shaft, and an enlarged tip.

Internally, the penis is cylindrical; the penile shaft consists of three columns of erectile tissue held together by strong fibrous tissue (Fig. 9.4):

• The corpus cavernosum is made up of two columns forming the major part of the dorsal (uppermost) and lateral (side) volumes of the penis.

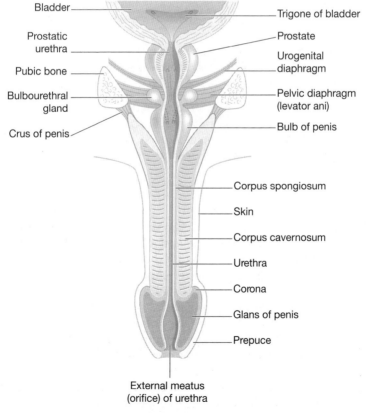

Bladder — Trigone of bladder
Prostatic urethra — Prostate
Pubic bone — Urogenital diaphragm
Bulbourethral gland — Pelvic diaphragm (levator ani)
Crus of penis — Bulb of penis
— Corpus spongiosum
— Skin
— Corpus cavernosum
— Urethra
— Corona
— Glans of penis
— Prepuce
External meatus (orifice) of urethra

**Figure 9.4**   Coronal schematic view of the penis.

- The corpus spongiosum forms the ventral (underside) portion, which expands over the distal end, forming the glans penis, and encases the urethra's proximal end, which is enlarged to form the bulb of the penis.
- The glans penis is a cone-shaped structure formed from corpus spongiosum; its lateral margins form a ridge of tissue known as the corona. The glans is well supplied with sensory receptors.

The male urethra is 20 cm long, commences at the bladder neck, and terminates at the urethral orifice on the glans penis. The urethra has three parts:

- The prostatic urethra runs through the prostate and expands into an area called the seminal colliculus, into which the seminal vesicle ducts also open.
- The membranous urethra lies between the apex of the prostate and the bulb of the penis, surrounded by a sphincter and perineal membrane.
- The spongy urethra passes through the bulb, the corpus spongiosum, and the glans penis; immediately before the external urethral orifice, the urethra expands to form the navicular fossa.

The skin of the penis, well supplied with sensory receptors, is a thin, loose skin that covers the penile shaft and includes a fold that extends to cover the glans penis. Called the prepuce (foreskin), this loose fold may be removed by circumcision.

## Oncology

Penile cancer is a rare disease and, when diagnosed early, is very curable. Unfortunately, the outlook worsens with later stage disease (III and IV). It is generally believed that a relationship exists between hygiene and cancer; this is demonstrated by populations that practice circumcision, such as orthodox Jews, in whom penile cancer is virtually unknown. About half of the males who have problems retracting their foreskin (phimosis) will go on to develop penile cancer, suggesting that hygiene and washing of the penis may be a good form of prevention. The coronal glands of the glans penis secrete a product called smegma, and if the glans beneath the foreskin is not regularly cleaned, a build-up of this secretion may lead to infection and may ultimately become carcinogenic.

Premalignant conditions, such as viral warts (a benign condition) and condyloma acuminatum (cauliflower-like warts on the perineum and penis), are caused by human papilloma virus (HPV) subtypes HPV6 and HPV11.

Penile carcinomas present almost entirely as squamous cell carcinomas that vary from well- to moderately differentiated. Penile carcinomas are usually seen in elderly men who are uncircumcised. The lesion presents as a warty, cauliflower growth that bleeds easily. Penile carcinomas can also present as a solid growth on the shaft, causing ulceration, or may grow insidiously under the foreskin. The lesions are usually slow-growing, and patients often delay diagnosis because of personal embarrassment. Malignant lesions can display a spectrum of changes from dysplasia to carcinoma in situ (also known as erythroplasia of Queyrat or Bowen's disease of the penis). These tumors are grouped as penile intraepithelial neoplasia, and many cases are now associated with HPV infection. The condition leads to invasive cancer unless treated intensively with local irradiation or 5-fluorouracil cream. These lesions can present as single or multiple flat, red glistening areas.

Clinically, these symptoms, warty growths on the glans sulcus or base of glans, are often present for over a year before a patient seeks medical help. An infection or bloody discharge can occur under the foreskin. If the lesion is visible, diagnosis is obvious. If phimosis hides it, the glans must be exposed by a dorsal slit in the prepuce or complete circumcision with biopsy. Inguinal nodes may be enlarged, suggesting spread or infection. Blood-borne metastases are rare and late. Staging is by the TNM classification (see Box 9.4 and Table 9.6).

### Treatment

If the tumor is carcinoma in situ, the treatment is local application of 5-fluorouracil cream. A relatively new therapy using Nd:YAG laser therapy has so far produced excellent control and possible cure while still preserving cosmetic appearance and sexual function, but it is still under clinical evaluation. Once the tumor becomes infiltrative, with or without local skin involvement, the choice of therapy is determined by tumor size, extent of infiltration, and the amount of normal tissue destruction. The options are amputation of the penis (partial or complete), external beam radiotherapy (including brachytherapy), and/or microscopically

---

**Box 9.4**   Staging of penile cancer—TNM definitions

**Primary tumor (T)**
TX: Primary tumor cannot be assessed
T0: No evidence of primary tumor
Tis: Carcinoma in situ
Ta: Non-invasive verrucous carcinoma
T1: Tumor invades subepithelial connective tissue
T2: Tumor invades corpus spongiosum or cavernosum
T3: Tumor invades urethra or prostrate
T4: Tumor invades other adjacent structures

**Regional lymph node involvement (N)**
NX: Regional lymph nodes cannot be assessed
N0: No regional lymph node metastasis
N1: Metastasis in a single superficial inguinal lymph node
N2: Metastasis in multiple or bilateral superficial inguinal lymph nodes
N3: Metastasis in deep or pelvic lymph node(s), unilateral or bilateral

**Distant metastasis (M)**
MX: Distant metastasis cannot be assessed
M0: No distant metastasis
M1: Distant metastasis

---

**Table 9.6**   Penile cancer—stage groups

| Stage | Primary tumor | Regional node involvement | Distant metastasis |
|-------|---------------|---------------------------|--------------------|
| 0     | Tis           | N0                        | M0                 |
|       | Ta            | N0                        | M0                 |
| I     | T1            | N0                        | M0                 |
| II    | T1            | N1                        | M0                 |
|       | T2            | N0                        | M0                 |
|       | T2            | N1                        | M0                 |
| III   | T1            | N2                        | M0                 |
|       | T2            | N2                        | M0                 |
|       | T3            | N0                        | M0                 |
|       | T3            | N1                        | M0                 |
|       | T3            | N2                        | M0                 |
| IV    | T4            | Any N                     | M0                 |
|       | Any T         | N3                        | M0                 |
|       | Any T         | Any N                     | M1                 |

controlled surgery. Because the outlook rapidly declines at later stages, patients are often entered into clinical trials. One trial is at present evaluating the use of radiosensitizers and/or chemotherapy as adjuvant therapy, and so far seems to be quite promising. Surgery involving amputation of part of or the whole penis is curative in 70% of patients if nodes are not involved, but patients are usually not enthusiastic about this form of treatment.

Radiotherapy (or brachytherapy) is commonly the treatment of choice, as it permits the penis to be conserved. However, since radiotherapy is a local treatment, control is poor if the tumor has deeply invaded the tissue. Superficial tumors treated early have a very high cure rate. In general, early stage penile cancer has a good prognosis. Unfortunately, at later stages the survival rates drop off rapidly.

## SELF-ASSESSMENT QUESTIONS

Answer true or false to the following. Answers are on page 244.

1. The testes are a pair of oval organs that initially develop high up on the anterior wall of the abdomen at about the level of the kidneys.
2. The spermatic cord is composed of a muscle, blood, lymph, nerve supply, and the vas deferens.
3. Within the testes are 200–300 compartments called lobules, which contain interstitial cells and 1–4 seminiferous tubules.
4. The routes of spread of cancer of both the testis and scrotum are the same.
5. The strongest risk factor associated with testicular cancer is carcinoma in situ.
6. Testicular cancer is the most common solid tumor in young men aged 15–39 years.
7. For sperm to develop normally they require to maintain a temperature 3°C below core body temperature.
8. 90–95% of testicular tumors are germ cell tumors; they are classified into two groups: seminoma and non-seminoma.
9. Treatment management of testicular cancer is based on whether the tumor is of a seminoma or non-seminoma type.
10. The prostate is a small organ which lies directly beneath the bladder.
11. The prostate gland is divided into three zones: peripheral, transitional, and caudal.
12. Classically, the symptoms of prostate cancer are very similar to those of benign hyperplasia of the prostate.
13. Cancer of the prostate is one of the most common cancers in males, accounting for about 30% of all new cancers diagnosed in males.
14. The most important factor associated with prostate cancer is the relatively high median age at diagnosis.
15. The majority of prostate tumors are adenocarcinomas.
16. The peripheral zone is the largest region of the prostate gland and is the zone where the majority of prostatic cancer arises.
17. Prostate-specific antigen (PSA) is produced only by the prostate and is a useful tumor marker.

18. A patient with prostate cancer with a high Gleason score is likely to experience a long, slow progression and may not develop any symptoms for 10 years or more.
19. Penile carcinomas are almost entirely adenocarcinomas.
20. It is generally believed that there is a relationship between hygiene and cancer of the penis.

# 10

# The female reproductive system (including breast)

The female reproductive system includes the pelvic organs (Fig. 10.1)—comprising the uterus, ovaries, vagina, and vulva—along with the breasts, which are classified as external accessory sex organs. The function of the female reproductive system is to produce ova (eggs), provide an environment for a fertilized egg to develop into a fetus, and to deliver the full-term baby during childbirth. To enable the reproductive organs to fulfill this function, hormones are produced by the ovaries to sustain this cycle of events. The function of the breasts is to provide nutrition for the

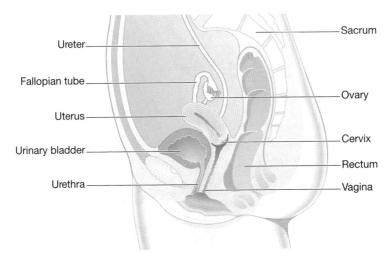

**Figure 10.1**   The female pelvis in sagittal section, showing relational anatomy.

newborn child in the form of milk; this function is also under the control of hormones.

## UTERUS

The normal uterus is the size of a medium pear and consists of three parts: the fundus, the body, and the cervix. The function of the uterus is to provide an environment for a fertilized egg to develop into a fetus. It is important to note that the cervix is not a separate anatomical organ but is the lower third of the uterus (the word cervix means neck). Lying in the pelvic cavity between the bladder in front and the rectum behind (see Fig. 10.1), the size and position of the uterus can vary depending on factors such as age, pregnancy, and other pelvic organ size. The uterus normally lies flexed over the superior surface of the bladder with the cervix pointing downwards and backwards, joining the vagina at right angles. It is not uncommon, however, for the uterus to tilt back-wards, and this is known as retroflexion.

The uterine wall has three layers: an outer serous layer (perimetrium), a middle muscular layer (myometrium), and the inner layer or endometrium (see Fig. 10.2). The perimetrium is part of the peritoneum that laterally forms the broad ligament. The myometrium has three layers of smooth muscle fibers, which

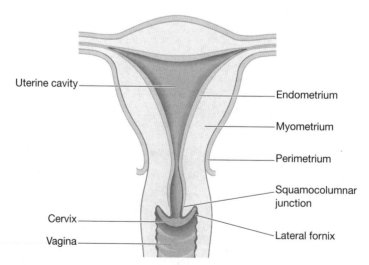

**Figure 10.2**   The uterus in section, showing the three layers.

produce coordinated contractions during childbirth to help delivery of the baby. The endometrium has two layers: a permanent layer called the stratum basalis and a surface layer called the stratum functionalis. This inner layer is composed of columnar epithelium which is in folds, forming numerous glands. The endometrium is under hormonal control and prepares to receive a fertilized egg each month. If fertilization does not occur, the outer stratum functionalis is removed during menstruation and is replaced by the stratum basalis.

The internal os at the inferior end of the uterus opens out into the cervical canal, which is constricted at its lower end, forming the external os that opens into the vagina (see Fig. 10.2). The cell type changes in this area from columnar to squamous epithelium and is known as the squamous-columnar (or squamocolumnar) junction. The cervix projects into the vaginal vault, and the area around this projection is known as the fornix. This projection into the vagina allows cervical smears to be done relatively easily.

# Oncology

Two different histological types of tumor occur in the uterus, distinguished not only by the different types of tissue, but also by very different (and often juxtaposed) causative factors associated with the presenting diseases. The two pathologies are those affecting the body of the uterus and those affecting the cervix.

### Carcinoma of the cervix

Carcinoma of the cervix is the second most common malignancy in women worldwide. It is mainly a disease of women in their 40s and 50s, but there is a trend towards higher rates of diagnosis in younger women. This trend is partly associated with the cervical screening program that is diagnosing more in-situ carcinoma rather than invasive carcinoma. Cervical cancer is more common in lower socio-economic groups and has a wide geographical variation, with Zimbabwe and South America having higher incidences than the UK and USA.

**Etiology**   There are a number of factors associated with carcinoma of the cervix, the major risk factor being human papilloma virus (HPV) infection. Other known risk factors include young age at first intercourse, a high number of sexual partners, and high parity (number of children). It is thought that these associated risk factors are linked to HPV, as this is transmitted during sexual activity. There is more than one type of HPV, which may explain why the number of sexual partners may increase the risk of developing carcinoma of the cervix. Another risk factor which has been linked to the development of carcinoma of the cervix is the prolonged use of oral contraceptives. This linkage could be due either to hormone manipulation or to the freedom of sexual activity without the risk of pregnancy afforded by oral contraceptives.

**General pathology** Macroscopically, carcinoma of the cervix appears as a proliferative growth or as an ulcer in the cervical region. The majority (90%) are of squamous cell carcinoma (SCC) type with a few adenocarcinomas. If the tumor is confined to the surface epithelium it is described as non-invasive. This non-invasive (sometimes referred to as pre-invasive) stage is described as CIN (cervical intraepithelial neoplasia). Thirty to forty percent of cases will progress to involve the submucosa, and the tumor is then termed frankly invasive. CIN is graded according to the degree of differentiation, the appearance of the cell nucleus, and the mitotic activity and has three levels: CIN I, II, and III. CIN III is sometimes referred to as severe dysplasia or carcinoma in situ.

The cervical screening programs in the UK and USA have proved very successful. Although the overall number of cervical carcinomas has not dropped, there is widespread, good evidence that the rate of decline in invasive cervical cancer and the associated rise in CIN is related to the intensity of screening. Around 4.5 million cervical smears are performed annually in the UK, and this is estimated to have reduced invasive carcinoma by 30%. Early diagnosis allows treatment to be given both early and successfully. In the UK cervical smears are recommended for sexually active women aged 20–64 and should be performed every 3 years. In the USA, screening is recommended for all sexually active women and for all women over the age of 18 annually, with increased time between tests after three normal results.

**Invasive carcinoma** Frankly invasive carcinoma, if untreated, will spread in all directions: to the adjoining tissues and organs of the pelvis, including the vaginal vault, the fornices and the endometrium, as well as laterally to the parametria, anteriorly to the bladder, and posteriorly to the rectum. Lymphatic spread is identified in 15% of stage I tumors, and blood-borne metastases can occur, primarily to the lungs, liver, and bone.

**Clinical features** Cervical cancer is often asymptomatic, particularly at an early (CIN) stage and is often diagnosed from routine cervical screening. Symptoms can include vaginal bleeding, particularly after intercourse, and vaginal discharge. These symptoms are not always picked up quickly, as irregular bleeding can be mistaken for menopausal symptoms by women in their 40s and 50s and not reported to the doctor.

**Investigations** Investigations include a full blood count to check for anemia following abnormal blood loss, routine biochemical tests to check liver function, and a chest X-ray to exclude lung metastases. Cervical biopsy and cytology are carried out to diagnose the malignancy histologically, and, if there is vaginal discharge, swabs will be taken to check for infection. Computed tomography (CT) scans of abdomen and pelvis are undertaken to assess the local extent of tumor and lymphatic involvement.

**Staging** Staging of cervical cancer is by the TNM and International Federation of Gynecology and Obstetrics (FIGO) systems, as outlined in Box 10.1 and Table 10.1.

**Treatment** Treatment for pre-invasive carcinoma is by laser surgery, loop electrosurgical excision procedure (LEEP), conization, or cryosurgery. All have excellent treatment outcomes of nearly 100% and leave the cervix competent. This is important in young women who wish to have children at a future date. More extensive treatment may leave the cervix incompetent, which means there may be problems carrying a pregnancy to full term.

For invasive carcinoma, surgery and radiotherapy, alone or in combination, are curative. Factors influencing the choice of treatment include age, the general condition of the patient, and the stage of the disease, along with the patient's own preference. Patients may have chemotherapy combined with these modalities to treat systematic disease if the pelvic nodes have been found to be positive.

*Surgery* For some cases of invasive cervical carcinoma, a radical hysterectomy, which includes removal of the entire uterus, ovaries, fallopian tubes, parametria, and the upper third of the vagina may be undertaken. This is known as Wertheim's hysterectomy. The addition of the upper third of the vagina to a normal hysterectomy is to prevent local recurrence from local invasion to the vagina. Removal of the ovaries and fallopian tubes (bilateral salpingo-oophorectomy) may not be required in early stage disease as tumors will rarely have spread this far. The advantage of sparing

---

**Box 10.1** Staging of cervical cancer—TNM and FIGO definitions

**Primary tumor (T) / FIGO stage**
- TX: Primary tumor cannot be assessed
- T0: No evidence of primary tumor
- Tis/0: Carcinoma in situ
- T1/I: Cervical carcinoma confined to uterus (disregard extension to corpus)
  —T1a/IA: Invasive carcinoma diagnosed only by microscopy. All macroscopically visible lesions, even with superficial invasion, are T1b/IB. Stromal invasion with a maximal depth of 5 mm measured from the base of the epithelium and a horizontal spread of 7 mm or less. Vascular space involvement, venous or lymphatic, does not affect the classification
    —T1a1/IA1: Measured stromal invasion 3 mm or less in depth and 7 mm or less in horizontal spread
    —T1a2/IA2: Measured stromal invasion more than 3 mm and not more than 5 mm, with a horizontal spread 7 mm or less
  —T1b/IB: Clinically visible lesion confined to the cervix or microscopic lesion greater than T1a2/IA2
    —T1b1/IB1: Clinically visible lesion 4 cm or less in greatest dimension
    —T1b2/IB2: Clinically visible lesion more than 4 cm in greatest dimension
- T2/II: Cervical carcinoma invades beyond uterus but not to pelvic wall or to the lower third of the vagina
  —T2a/IIA: Tumor without parametrial involvement
  —T2b/IIB: Tumor with parametrial involvement
- T3/III: Tumor extends to the pelvic wall and/or involves the lower third of the vagina and/or causes hydronephrosis or non-functioning kidney
  —T3a/IIIA: Tumor involves lower third of the vagina, no extension to pelvic wall
  —T3b/IIIB: Tumor extends to pelvic wall and/or causes hydronephrosis or non-functioning kidney
- T4/IV: Tumor invades mucosa of the bladder or rectum, and/or extends beyond true pelvis

**Regional lymph node involvement (N)**
- NX: Regional lymph nodes cannot be assessed
- N0: No regional lymph node metastasis
- N1: Regional lymph node metastasis

**Distant metastasis (M)**
- MX: Distant metastasis cannot be assessed
- M0: No distant metastasis
- M1: Distant metastasis

Adapted from Benedet JL et al. Carcinoma of the cervix uteri. *J Epidemiol Biostat* 2001; 6(1):5–44.

---

the ovaries is that hormone function will remain. This will not be the case if radiotherapy is used, since the ovaries cannot be spared and irradiation will cause loss of hormone function and fertility.

*Radiotherapy* Radical radiotherapy for early stage disease results in long-term survival rates similar to those for surgery but

**Table 10.1**  Cervical cancer—stage groups

| Stage | Primary tumor | Regional node involvement | Distant metastasis |
|---|---|---|---|
| 0 | Tis | N0 | M0 |
| I | T1 | N0 | M0 |
| IA | T1a | N0 | M0 |
| IA1 | T1a1 | N0 | M0 |
| IA2 | T1a2 | N0 | M0 |
| IB | T1b | N0 | M0 |
| IB1 | T1b1 | N0 | M0 |
| IB2 | T1b2 | N0 | M0 |
| II | T2 | N0 | M0 |
| IIA | T2a | N0 | M0 |
| IIB | T2b | N0 | M0 |
| III | T3 | N0 | M0 |
| IIIA | T3a | N0 | M0 |
| IIIB | T1 | N1 | M0 |
|  | T2 | N1 | M0 |
|  | T3a | N1 | M0 |
|  | T3b | Any N | M0 |
| IVA | T4 | Any N | M0 |
| IVB | Any T | Any N | M1 |

there may be greater morbidity because of the side effects of radiation on normal tissues. It is, however, an option for younger women who refuse radical surgery. Postoperative radiotherapy following a Wertheim's hysterectomy can be used where the excision margins are not clear of tumor and pelvic nodes are found to be positive.

Radical radiotherapy normally requires a combination of internal (brachytherapy) and external irradiation. Brachytherapy is delivered by means of the intracavitary insertion of a uterine tube and ovoids containing a radioactive source that can deliver a high central dose to the cervix. If the pelvic lymph nodes are involved, the pelvis is treated with external radiotherapy.

*Palliative treatment*  Palliative radiotherapy can be given for advanced local disease to control bleeding and pelvic pain.

*Hormone replacement therapy*  Cervical cancer is not hormone dependent; therefore, hormone manipulation is not useful. However, following radical treatment for young women, hormone replacement therapy should be considered because of the loss of ovarian function.

*Prognosis*  The outcome is closely related to the stage at presentation, with 5-year survival of around 80% for stages I and II, 40% for stage III, and 15% for stage IV. For CIN, the treatment is almost always curative, which proves the need for early diagnosis.

### Cancer of the body of the uterus (corpus uteri)

Cancer of the body of the uterus is normally referred to as endometrial carcinoma because it affects the inner lining of the body of the uterus, the endometrium. Tumors arise mainly from the glandular epithelium (adenocarcinomas) and are therefore different in origin from those arising at the cervix. Endometrial carcinoma accounts for approximately 4% of all cancers in women and is mainly a disease of postmenopausal women. There is less geographical variation than in cervical carcinoma but the disease is rare in Japan compared with Europe and the USA.

**Etiology**  The predominant risk factor for endometrial carcinoma is related to hormone activity. Endometrial carcinoma occurs more commonly in women who have no children (nulliparous) or few children. Other risk factors are diabetes, obesity, and cardiovascular disease. These risk factors are linked by excessive stimulation of estrogens, causing overgrowth of the endometrium and subsequent malignancy. There is a similar link with women on hormone replacement therapy and those prescribed tamoxifen for carcinoma of the breast, although the benefits of these treatments must be considered along with the associated risk. A further factor associating this disease with a hormonal influence is the higher incidence in women who have an early menarche and late menopause. There is no association with age of the woman at first birth, unlike breast carcinoma (described later in this chapter).

**Pathology**  Macroscopically, tumors arising within the uterine cavity may be polypoid or diffuse multifocal growths. They arise from the glandular epithelium of the endometrium, and microscopically they are predominantly adenocarcinomas, the majority being well differentiated. Sarcomas may arise from the muscular layer of the uterus but are rare.

If untreated, local spread can occur, as in cervical cancer, to the adjoining tissues and organs of the pelvis. Local invasion tends to be to the myometrium and cervix, but the fallopian tubes and ovaries can also be involved if the primary is nearer the fundus of the uterus. Spread to the bladder and rectum is less common with endometrial carcinoma than with cervical carcinoma, which may be due to the barrier formed by the serous layer of the uterine body, which does not extend down to the cervical area. If the primary occurs around the endocervix, it may not be possible to differentiate whether it is an endometrial or a cervical primary.

The incidence of lymphatic involvement is related to the depth of invasion of the myometrium, and this occurs less in well differentiated than in poorly differentiated tumors. Late spread via the blood may occur to the lungs and bones.

**Clinical features**   The classic presentation of endometrial carcinoma is irregular bleeding, in particular postmenopausal bleeding. As in cervical carcinoma this may not be reported early, as it may be thought of as a normal menopausal symptom. Endometrial carcinoma may also be detected as an incidental finding during cervical screening.

**Investigations**   A full blood count should be done to check for anemia resulting from chronic blood loss. For histological diagnosis a hysteroscopy and biopsy will be done under general anesthetic. A chest X-ray may be done to exclude metastases, along with a CT scan to assess local spread and lymph node status.

**Staging**   Staging is by the FIGO and TNM classifications as outlined in Box 10.2 and Table 10.2.

**Treatment**

*Surgery*   The main form of treatment for endometrial carcinoma is a total hysterectomy with removal of the ovaries (bilateral salpingo-oophorectomy). A Wertheim's hysterectomy is performed if there is cervical involvement (stage II), which, as in cervical carcinoma, additionally involves removal of the upper third of the vagina.

*Radiotherapy*   Postoperative radiotherapy can be given following hysterectomy for stage I disease, depending on the risk factors for local and distant dissemination, such as depth of myometrial invasion. Well differentiated tumors with minimal myometrial invasion may receive brachytherapy by means of vaginal irradiation only; moderately or poorly differentiated tumors and those invading the mid- to outer third of myometrium should have both external and intravaginal treatment.

Radical radiotherapy can be given to those patients who are not suitable for surgery, either because of concurrent disease or inoperable tumors. This is usually external beam treatment followed by intracavitary treatment to the uterus and upper vagina. Palliative radiotherapy can be given for locally advanced tumors and painful bony metastases.

**Box 10.2** Staging of endometrial carcinoma—TNM and FIGO definitions

**Primary tumor (T) / FIGO stage**
- TX: Primary tumor cannot be assessed
- T0: No evidence of primary tumor
- Tis/0: Carcinoma in situ
- T1/I: Tumor confined to corpus uteri
  —T1a/IA: Tumor limited to endometrium
  —T1b/IB: Tumor invades less than one half of the myometrium
  —T1c/IC: Tumor invades one half or more of the myometrium
- T2: Tumor invades cervix but does not extend beyond uterus
  —T2a/IIA: Endocervical glandular involvement only
  —T2b/IIB: Cervical stromal invasion
- T3: Local and/or regional spread as in T3a, T3b, and/or N1
  —T3a/IIIA: Tumor involves serosa and/or adnexa (direct extension or metastasis) and/or cancer cells in ascites or peritoneal washings
  —T3b/IIIB: Vaginal involvement (direct extension or metastasis)
- T4/IVA: Tumor invades bladder mucosa and/or bowel mucosa

**Regional lymph node involvement (N)**
- NX: Regional lymph nodes cannot be assessed
- N0: No regional lymph node metastasis
- N1/IIIC: Regional lymph node metastasis to pelvic and/or para-aortic lymph nodes

**Distant metastasis (M)**
- MX: Distant metastasis cannot be assessed
- M0: No distant metastasis
- M1/IVB: Distant metastasis (excluding metastasis to vagina, pelvic serosa, or adnexa; including metastasis to intra-abdominal lymph nodes other than para-aortic, and/or inguinal lymph nodes

Adapted from Creasman WT et al. Carcinoma of the corpus uteri. *J Epidemiol Biostat* 2001; 6(1):45–86.

*Hormonal treatment*  Endometrial carcinoma is hormone dependent, and locally advanced or metastatic disease responds to progesterones. Response rates are only 20–30%, but this treatment may be useful for palliation of symptomatic metastases.

**Prognosis**  The prognosis overall is good, as the majority of patients present with stage I disease. Around 90% 5-year survival for stage I disease can be achieved. For advanced disease, 5-year survival rates fall to 65% for stage II and 35% for stage III.

# OVARY

Each ovary (Fig. 10.3) is the size and shape of a large almond. The ovaries are located below and behind the uterine tubes at the side of the uterus and are attached to the uterus by a ligament. The end

**Table 10.2** Endometrial carcinoma—stage groups

| Stage | Primary tumor | Regional node involvement | Distant metastasis |
| --- | --- | --- | --- |
| 0 | Tis | N0 | M0 |
| I | T1 | N0 | M0 |
| IA | T1a | N0 | M0 |
| IB | T1b | N0 | M0 |
| IC | T1c | N0 | M0 |
| II | T2 | N0 | M0 |
| IIA | T2a | N0 | M0 |
| IIB | T2b | N0 | M0 |
| III | T3 | N0 | M0 |
| IIIA | T3a | N0 | M0 |
| IIIB | T3b | N1 | M0 |
| IIIC | T1 | N1 | M0 |
| | T2 | N1 | M0 |
| | T3 | Any N | M0 |
| IVA | T4 | Any N | M0 |
| IVB | Any T | Any N | M1 |

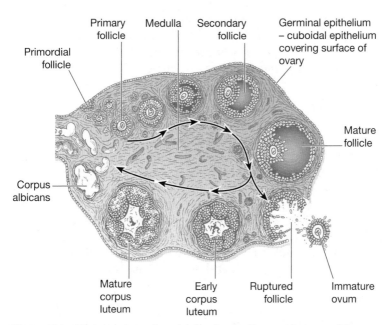

**Figure 10.3** The ovary in section, showing the developmental stages of the ovarian cycle.

of the uterine (fallopian) tube curves over the ovary but is not attached to it. The ovary has two functions: ovulation and hormone secretion. The ovary is covered by a layer of germinal epithelium, although this is perhaps misleading as it is not the tissue that develops the ova. The ova are found in structures called ovarian follicles that are embedded in connective tissue toward the center of the ovary. These follicles consist of an oocyte surrounded by specialized hormone-secreting cells (granulosa). The oocytes are under the influence of follicle-stimulating hormone (FSH), which is produced by the pituitary gland. The oocytes start to grow each month following puberty. FSH also stimulates the secretion of estrogen by the follicles. Other hormones then become involved to stimulate ovulation and further production of estrogen along with progesterone. This monthly menstrual cycle is in three phases. In the first, or menstrual phase, the inner lining of the endometrium is lost; during this phase the ovarian follicles also begin their development. The second phase or preovulatory stage is when the follicles produce estrogens to stimulate the repair of the endometrium and the follicle becomes ready for ovulation. Ovulation occurs when an immature ovum is released into the pelvic cavity. The final stage is the postovulatory stage when the endometrium starts to thicken in preparation for fertilization and implantation of the embryo. If this does not occur, the cycle repeats itself and menstruation and follicular development start again.

## Oncology

Ovarian cancer is a disease that kills more women than any other gynecologic malignancy. Even with aggressive treatment, the survival rates are poor. Early detection would save lives, but the manifestation of the disease makes this in itself problematic. There are around 6000 new cases of ovarian cancer in the UK each year, accounting for 4% of all women's cancer, and over 4000 deaths per year. There is a similar incidence in the USA, accounting for around 25 000 cases and 14 000 deaths per year. In Japan, there is a low incidence, but in Japanese immigrants to the USA the ovarian cancer incidence approaches that of American women.

### Etiology

Ovarian carcinoma tends to occur in women over 40 years. Although the etiology is generally unknown, there is a higher incidence in nulliparous women and higher socio-economic groups. There is increasing evidence of genetic factors (5% of cases), with links to the breast cancer gene *BRCA1*, as well as blood group A. As in endometrial carcinoma, ovarian carcinoma is related to hormones, and the risk of ovarian carcinoma decreases with the number of pregnancies.

## Pathology

There is a wide variety of tumor cell types, 90% of which arise from the surface epithelium. Of these, 10% are borderline malignancy with no invasion, 1–2% arise from germ cells, which are commoner in young women, and 2% from specialized hormone-producing cells (see Table 10.3). Secondary tumors can also occur in the ovary from carcinoma of the uterus, breast, or gastrointestinal tract (Krukenberg tumors).

## Clinical features

Ovarian tumors tend to grow slowly and silently for a long time and, as a result, they are usually at an advanced stage at diagnosis. Sixty percent will have spread outside the pelvis at presentation,

**Table 10.3** Histological types of ovarian cancer

| Histological types | Cytological variations |
| --- | --- |
| Epithelial tumors (92%) | Serous tumors (42%)—fluid content resembles serum; often bilateral<br>Mucinous tumors (12%)—mucin produced by cells; often multicystic<br>Clear cell carcinoma (6%)<br>Endometrioid carcinoma (15%)—arising from endometriosis<br>Undifferentiated carcinoma (17%) |
| Germ cell tumors (6%) | Dysgerminoma—rare; analogous to seminoma of the testis<br>Teratoma—mostly benign (unlike its male counterpart); differentiate to the various embryonal layers<br>Choriocarcinoma<br>Yolk sac tumor |
| Hormone-producing cell tumors (2%) | Granulosa cell tumors—secrete estrogen; cause early puberty in children and excess feminism in adults<br>Androblastomas—rare, benign; may produce male hormones with resultant hair growth and deep voice |

and some tumors, particularly benign tumors, can attain sizes resembling an advanced pregnancy and eventually cause pressure symptoms. In hormone-producing tumors, the first symptoms may be from the action of the hormones, rather than from the growth itself.

Lymphatic spread to the para-aortic nodes and blood-borne metastases to liver and lungs occur late. Most tumors are cystic and spread to the outer peritoneal surface, or the cyst ruptures into the peritoneal cavity. Cells become attached to or invade adjacent structures, including the fallopian tubes, uterus, large and small bowel, and bladder. Deposits from ruptured tumors may seed far and wide on peritoneal surfaces as high up as the diaphragm.

### Investigations

Routine tests are often unremarkable, although in advanced cases there may be electrolyte disturbance from intestinal obstruction or ureteric obstruction causing renal failure. A laparotomy is necessary to assess the extent of the disease. Ultrasound of ovaries and liver, along with CT scan of abdomen and pelvis, can demonstrate primary tumor, lymph nodes, and liver metastases if present.

The tumor marker CA125 is a valuable blood marker for ovarian cancer; normal levels are in the range 1–35 U/ml. Women with levels above 30 U/ml are thought to be at increased risk of having ovarian cancer, but it is not specific to ovarian cancer and the level is not always elevated in the presence of ovarian cancer. CA125 is not yet being used as a screening method, although trials are being done, but it can be useful in monitoring response to treatment.

### Staging

Staging for ovarian cancer is by the TNM and FIGO systems as outlined in Box 10.3 and Table 10.4.

### Treatment

**Surgery**   The primary treatment for ovarian carcinoma is surgery. All patients with operable disease should have a laparotomy and a total abdominal hysterectomy with bilateral salpingo-oophorectomy. Both ovaries are removed, as a significant number of tumors are bilateral or carry the risk of metastatic disease to the contralateral ovary. It may be possible to remove only the affected

---

**Box 10.3**  Staging of ovarian cancer—TNM and FIGO definitions

**Primary tumor (T) / FIGO**
- TX: Primary tumor cannot be assessed
- T0: No evidence of primary tumor
- T1/I: Tumor limited to the ovaries (one or both)
  - —T1a/IA: Tumor limited to one ovary; capsule intact, no tumor on ovarian surface, no malignant cells in ascites or peritoneal washings[a]
  - —T1b/IB: Tumor limited to both ovaries; capsule intact, no tumor on ovarian surface, no malignant cells in ascites or peritoneal washings[a]
  - —T1c/IC: Tumor limited to one or both ovaries with any of the following: capsule ruptured, tumor on ovarian surface, malignant cells in ascites or peritoneal washings[a]
- T2/II: Tumor involves one or both ovaries with pelvic extension and/or implants
  - —T2a/IIA: Extension and/or implants on the uterus and/or tube(s); no malignant cells in ascites or peritoneal washings[a]
  - —T2b/IIB: Extension to and/or implants on other pelvic tissues; no malignant cells in ascites or peritoneal washings[a]
  - —T2c/IIC: Pelvic extension and/or implants (T2a or T2b) with malignant cells in ascites or peritoneal washings[a]
- T3/III: Tumor involves one or both ovaries with microscopically confirmed peritoneal metastasis outside pelvis
  - —T3a/IIIA: Microscopic peritoneal metastasis beyond pelvis (no macroscopic tumor)
  - —T3b/IIIB: Macroscopic peritoneal metastasis beyond pelvis 2 cm or less in greatest dimension
  - —T3c/IIIC: Peritoneal metastasis beyond the pelvis more than 2 cm in greatest dimension

**Regional lymph node involvement (N)**
- NX: Regional lymph nodes cannot be assessed
- N0: No regional lymph node metastasis
- N1: Regional lymph node metastasis

**Distant metastasis (M)**
- MX: Distant metastasis cannot be assessed
- M0: No distant metastasis
- M1: Distant metastasis (excluding peritoneal metastasis)

---

[a] The presence of non-malignant ascites is not classified. The presence of ascites does not affect staging unless malignant cells are present.
Adapted from Heintz AP et al. Carcinoma of the ovary. *J Epidemiol Biostat* 2001; 6(1):107–138.

---

ovary in young women, as long as the tumor is confirmed to be unilateral, well differentiated, and mucinous, and the peritoneum is found to be negative. The patient must be kept under close surveillance, especially if pregnancy is to be considered. Following surgery, other forms of treatment may be given, depending on the stage of the disease. Stage I disease with normal postoperative CT scan and

**Table 10.4** Ovarian cancer—stage groups

| Stage | Primary tumor | Regional node involvement | Distant metastasis |
|-------|---------------|---------------------------|--------------------|
| I | T1 | N0 | M0 |
| IA | T1a | N0 | M0 |
| IB | T1b | N0 | M0 |
| IC | T1c | N0 | M0 |
| II | T2 | N0 | M0 |
| IIA | T2a | N0 | M0 |
| IIB | T2b | N0 | M0 |
| IIC | T2c | N0 | M0 |
| III | T3 | N0 | M0 |
| IIIA | T3a | N0 | M0 |
| IIIB | T3b | N0 | M0 |
| IIIC | T3c | N0 | M0 |
| | Any T | N1 | M0 |
| IV | Any T | Any N | M1 |

normal CA125 levels requires no further treatment other than close observation. Patients with stages II and III disease should have chemotherapy. Stage IV disease with soft tissue metastases has a poor prognosis.

**Radiotherapy**    Radiotherapy is not a suitable option for radical treatment of ovarian carcinoma because the whole abdomen would have to be included in the treatment area, and side effects of treatment would prevent a radical dose from being given.

**Palliative treatment**    Chemotherapy can be used for relapse, although, if the relapse is within 1 year, ovarian cancers tend not to respond to chemotherapy. Radiotherapy can be used for symptomatic pelvic masses, vaginal bleeding, and bony metastases.

### Prognosis

Overall, prognosis is poor because of the late presentation of the disease. Five-year survival for stage I tumors can be 95% if surgery has been adequate, and up to 70% for stage II. Five-year survival drops to 20% for stage III and less than 5% for stage IV.

## VAGINA AND VULVA

## Vaginal cancer

Primary tumors of the vagina are rare, accounting for 1–2% of gynecologic malignancies. Most tumors arising in the vagina

**Box 10.4** Staging of carcinoma of the vagina—TNM and FIGO definitions

**Primary tumor (T) / FIGO stage**
- TX: Primary tumor cannot be assessed
- T0: No evidence of primary tumor
- Tis/0: Carcinoma in situ
- T1/I: Tumor confined to vaginal canal
- T2/II: Tumor invades subvaginal/paravaginal tissues but not to pelvic wall[a]
- T3/III: Tumor extends to pelvic wall[a]
- T4/IV: Tumor invades mucosa of the bladder or rectum and/or rectum and/or extends beyond the true pelvis

**Regional lymph node involvement (N)**
- NX: Regional nodes cannot be assessed
- N0: No regional lymph node metastasis
- N1: Pelvic or inguinal lymph node metastasis

**Distant metastasis (M)**
- MX: Distant metastasis cannot be assessed
- M0: No distant metastasis
- M1: Distant metastasis

[a] Pelvic wall is defined as the muscle, fascia, associated neurovascular structures, or skeletal portions of the bony pelvis.
Adapted from Beller U et al. Carcinoma of the vagina. *J Epidemiol Biostat* 2001; 6(1):141–152.

**Table 10.5** Vaginal carcinoma—stage groups

| Stage | Primary tumor | Regional node involvement | Distant metastasis |
|---|---|---|---|
| 0 | Tis | N0 | M0 |
| I | T1 | N0 | M0 |
| II | T2 | N0 | M0 |
| III | T1–T3 | N1 | M0 |
|  | T3 | N0 | M0 |
| IVA | T4 | Any N | M0 |
| IVB | Any T | Any N | M1 |

are secondary deposits from the cervix, uterus, rectum, or ovary. Most occur in patients aged 60 years or over. Most tumors occur in the upper vagina; approximately 90% are SCC and 10% are adenocarcinomas. It may be difficult to differentiate between a vaginal or cervical primary in some cases, and biopsy will be required to confirm diagnosis. Vaginal bleeding tends to be the most common symptom.

Box 10.4 shows the TNM and FIGO definitions for staging vaginal cancer; Table 10.5 shows stage groups. Treatment is by either

---

**Box 10.5** Staging of carcinoma of the vulva—TNM and FIGO definitions

**Primary tumor (T) / FIGO stage**
- TX: Primary tumor cannot be assessed
- T0: No evidence of primary tumor
- Tis/O: Carcinoma in situ (pre-invasive carcinoma)
- T1/I: Tumor confined to vulva and/or peritoneum, 2 cm or less in greatest dimension
  —T1a/IA: Tumor confined to the vulva and/or perineum, 2 cm or less in greatest dimension, and with stromal invasion no greater than 1 mm[a]
  —T1b/IB: Tumor confined to the vulva and/or perineum, 2 cm or less in greatest dimension, and with stromal invasion greater than 1 mm[a]
- T2/II: Tumor confined to vulva and/or peritoneum, more than 2 cm in greatest dimension
- T3/III: Tumor of any size with adjacent spread to the lower urethra and/or vagina or anus
- T4/IVA: Tumor invades any of the following: upper urethral mucosa, bladder mucosa, rectal mucosa; or is fixed to the pubic bone

**Regional lymph node involvement (N) / FIGO stage**
- NX: Regional nodes cannot be assessed
- N0: No regional lymph node metastasis
- N1/IIIA: Unilateral regional lymph node metastasis
- N2/IVA: Bilateral regional lymph node metastasis

**Distant metastasis (M) / FIGO stage**
- MX: Distant metastasis cannot be assessed
- M0: No distant metastasis
- M1/IVB: Distant metastasis (including pelvic lymph node metastasis)

---

[a] The depth of invasion is defined as the measurement of the tumor from the epithelial–stromal junction of the adjacent most superficial dermal papilla to the deepest point of invasion.
Adapted from Beller U et al. Carcinoma of the vulva. *J Epidemiol Biostat* 2001; 6(1):153–174.

---

interstitial or intracavitary radiotherapy, with prognosis ranging from 75% 5-year survival at stage I to 20% for stage III.

## Vulvar cancer

Vulvar cancer is rare, predominantly affecting elderly women. There is an association with viral infections such as herpes simplex and human papilloma virus. Tumors are exophytic or ulcerative and may have an associated leukoplakia. Virtually all are squamous cell carcinomas. Symptoms include vulvar itching (70%), discharge, and bleeding.

Box 10.5 shows TNM and FIGO definitions for staging vulvar cancer; Table 10.6 shows stage groups. Surgery is the treatment of

**Table 10.6** Vulvar carcinoma—stage groups

| Stage | Primary tumor | Regional node involvement | Distant metastasis |
|---|---|---|---|
| 0 | Tis | N0 | M0 |
| I | T1 | N0 | M0 |
| IA | T1a | N0 | M0 |
| IB | T1b | N0 | M0 |
| II | T2 | N0 | M0 |
| III | T1 | N1 | M0 |
| | T2 | N1 | M0 |
| | T3 | N0 | M0 |
| | T3 | N1 | M0 |
| IVA | T1 | N2 | M0 |
| | T2 | N2 | M0 |
| | T3 | N2 | M0 |
| | T4 | Any N | M0 |
| IVB | Any T | Any N | M1 |

choice, along with regional node dissection to prevent unsalvageable recurrence. Radiotherapy may be used postoperatively both locally and to the lymphatics. Prognosis is good if lymphatics are not involved, with a 5-year survival of up to 80%, but this drops to below 50% in cases with lymphatic involvement.

# BREAST

The breasts, which are external accessory sex organs, lie on the anterior chest wall, attached to the pectoral muscles by a layer of connective tissue. Adult female breasts are composed of glandular, adipose (fatty), and fibrous tissue (see Fig. 10.4). Glandular tissue comprises 15–20 lobes in each breast, which are further divided into lobules composed of secretory alveoli arranged around small ducts or ductules (see Fig. 10.4a). These small ductules unite to form one lactiferous duct for each lobe, which converge at the nipple, opening at individual orifices on the surface of the nipple. Fibrous tissue known as Cooper's ligaments supports the lobules, with adipose tissue lying over the gland and between the lobes. The size of the breast is related to the amount of adipose tissue, not the amount of glandular tissue, and therefore size does not relate to functional ability.

Until puberty, both males and females have small amounts of breast tissue consisting of a few ducts. Breast development in the female occurs at puberty and is controlled by the female

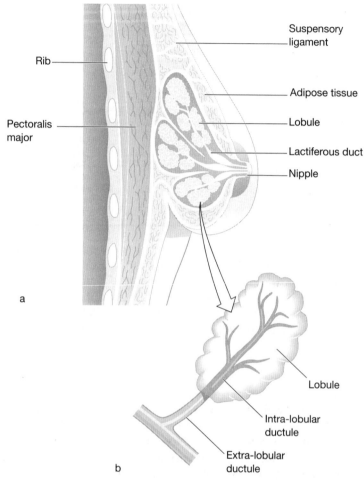

**Figure 10.4** (a) Sagittal section through the female breast; (b) terminal duct lobular unit.

hormones estrogen and progesterone. Estrogen is responsible for stimulating duct growth and progesterone for stimulating the development of the alveoli and secreting cells. In males, testosterone production prevents further growth development. The function of the female breast is secretion of milk via the lactiferous ducts and nipple.

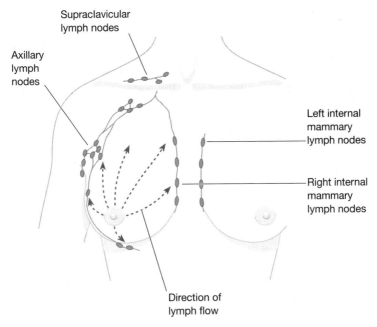

**Figure 10.5** Lymphatic drainage of the right breast.

From an oncology perspective, the lymphatic drainage of the breast is critically important, as spread of the disease and prognosis are directly related to lymphatic involvement. Two sets of lymphatic vessels drain the breast: those that originate in the skin and those that originate in the breast itself, including the nipple. Those in the skin form a cutaneous lymphatic plexus that connects with breast tissue lymphatics via the subareolar plexus under the nipple. The majority of breast lymph eventually drains to the axillary lymph nodes, with additional drainage to the supraclavicular nodes and to the internal mammary (also known as 'parasternal') nodes (Fig. 10.5). Lymphatic spread from one breast to the other can occur via either the superficial or breast tissue lymphatics.

## Oncology

Breast cancer is the commonest form of malignancy in women in the western world, accounting for around 30% of all cancers in women. It is estimated that one in nine women will develop breast cancer at some point in her life, although it mainly affects women aged 40–70 years. Incidence increases with age, and is rare below 30 years of age. The incidence of breast cancer is rising, with over 39 000 cases per year in the UK in 2002 compared with 33 000 in 1997. Male breast cancer is rare and accounts for only 1% of all breast cancers. There is a wide demographic difference in the incidence of breast cancer, with a high incidence in the western world compared with Japan, but daughters and granddaughters of Japanese immigrants have rates approaching that of the indigenous population.

## Etiology

The etiology of breast cancer is unknown in most cases but there are a number of predisposing factors. Most have a hormonal influence as a common factor, as well as familial and genetic links. There is also an increased risk of malignancy associated with benign breast disease and exposure to radiation.

**Risk factors** The breast is continuously under hormonal influence, and breast tissue does not fully mature until after the woman has undergone a full-term pregnancy, when the body has undergone its full hormone cycle. There are many factors that link breast cancer with a hormonal cause. There is an increased incidence in women who start menarche early with an associated late menopause and therefore have a longer time when estrogens are active within the body. Having no children, or having them later in life, also has been shown to be a risk factor and may be related to the lack, or late maturation of the breast tissue. The use of contraceptive pills and hormone replacement therapy can increase the risk of breast cancer if used long-term, although it is thought that hormone replacement therapy probably promotes the growth of an existing tumor rather than initiating malignant change. Hormone replacement therapy also has many benefits for women's health, including a protective function against osteoporosis, and it is therefore important that the risks and benefits are discussed on an individual basis.

Diet and obesity are also known risk factors in the development of breast cancer. Premenopausal women have a reduced risk if they have a high body mass index or gain weight during adult life, whereas in postmenopausal women there is an increased risk with high body mass index. This association is greater with increasing age and years after menopause. The reason is thought to be increased estrogen production from adipose tissue. Decreasing fat in the diet has been shown to decrease estrogen concentrations. Smoking also has been linked to the development of breast cancer, especially when started at a young age. This is related to immature breast tissue at this age, which is more susceptible to damage from chemical carcinogens. Risk of breast cancer also increases in women whose first-line relatives (mother, sister, or daughter) are diagnosed with breast cancer under the age of 40 years. Risk increases if two or more relatives from the same side of the family are diagnosed with breast cancer or if several relatives on the same side of the family are diagnosed with ovarian cancer.

There are probably several genes that can increase the risk of breast cancer: testing is available at present for *BRCA1* and *BRCA2*, and is offered to women in high-risk groups. If a woman carries either gene, the risk of developing breast cancer is over 80% by the age of 55 years. If the results of testing are positive, management options fall broadly into three groups. Each option should be discussed in depth with the patient, together with genetic counseling:

- regular screening (mammography), which increases the chance of cancer being detected
- surgery to remove both breasts followed by reconstructive surgery
- participation in a prevention trial, such as the use of tamoxifen and screening.

Less than 10% of women have a family history of breast cancer, and there is an independent chance unrelated to genetics that two or more women will be affected if they come from a large family. Methods of ascertaining exposure to estrogen are being investigated which may define the risk of developing breast cancer, particularly in high-risk groups. These are: cytological screening to determine plasma estrogen concentration, breast density tests, and bone mineral density tests.

Because of the increasing incidence of breast cancer and the apparent multitude of risk factors, models have been developed which attempt to calculate an individual's lifetime risk of developing breast cancer. These are not 100% reliable, as they tend to overpredict the risk for young women and do not always take into account all the factors which could be involved, therefore giving false results. What is important is that women are 'breast aware' and self-examine their breasts to detect changes early.

*Clinical features*

Breast tumors are often found by the patient or her partner as a painless lump in the breast. It is more common in the left breast, with 1–2% bilateral (synchronous) at the time of diagnosis and 7–8% subsequently developing a tumor in the other breast (metachronous). Increasingly, smaller tumors are being found through the breast screening program, although it has not been as successful in detecting early curable disease as the cervical screening program. This is due partly to mammography not being as specific in young breast tissue, which is dense, as it is in less dense postmenopausal breast tissue. At present, the screening program is primarily for women over 50 years of age, but recent evidence suggests that the minimum age could be reduced to 40 years. Other features of the disease, if not picked up early, are inversion of the nipple, distortion of overlying skin, inflammation of all or part of the breast, and fungation if left very late.

*Pathology*

Breast disease may be benign, premalignant (in situ), or malignant (invasive). Benign disease includes cysts, fibroadenomas, and papillomas; premalignant disease occurs in the ducts and lobes and is referred to as either ductal carcinoma in situ (DCIS) or lobular carcinoma in situ (LCIS). 'In situ' refers to the fact that the malignant cells are confined to the ducts or lobes. In-situ disease has the potential to become invasive, but how this change happens is unknown. Malignant tumors develop mainly from the glandular tissue (ducts and lobes) and are therefore adenocarcinomas.

The rate of diagnosis of DCIS has increased since the breast screening programs became active, but DCIS still accounts for only 15% of cases detected by mammography. There is a substantial risk of progression to invasive carcinoma, with an average delay of 7 years. LCIS, on the other hand, does not show up on mammograms and is often diagnosed by chance when a breast lump is biopsied. It is more common in premenopausal women than DCIS. LCIS has an increased associated risk of bilateral breast disease.

Invasive adenocarcinomas are classified according to the cell type as 'no special type' or special type, which includes tubular, mucoid, cribriform, papillary, medullary, and classic lobular. Inflammatory breast carcinoma, in which the breast becomes enlarged and warm, can also occur.

Histological grading of breast cancer is important, as it determines the management of the patient and correlates with local recurrence rate as well as the overall prognosis of the disease. Grading is based on three factors: nuclear pleomorphism, mitotic activity, and the degree of glandular formation. It is imperative that a histological diagnosis be made, as this, along with the TNM staging (see Box 10.6 and Table 10.7), is important in management decisions for the patient. As previously mentioned, lymphatic spread is an important aspect of the diagnosis and prognosis of breast cancer. Sampling and histological assessment of the axillary nodes also must be considered when patient management decisions are being made. Clinical examination alone will not always give a true picture of axillary node involvement: 30% of clinically palpable nodes are free of disease, and 30% considered free of disease are histologically positive. The breast can be divided into five areas anatomically (see Fig. 10.6). If the initial tumor is in the inner quadrants and there is lymphatic spread to the axillary nodes, there is a higher risk of the internal mammary nodes also being involved than if the tumor is in the outer quadrants. Breast cancer also spreads via the blood to the bones, liver, lungs, and brain.

Assessment of pathological lymph node status can also be enhanced by the use of staining techniques such as H&E (hematoxylin and eosin) staining for microscope slide making, IHC (immunohistochemical) marker staining, or molecular testing. This enhances the N classification as shown in Box 10.7.

### Treatment

Treatment for breast cancer has been and still is being researched. Historically, treatment was by surgery, which involved a radical mastectomy and axillary clearance. Unfortunately, women still died of metastatic disease even though they had undergone such radical treatment. Work then began on treating breast cancer as a systemic disease, which in the majority of cases is likely to have spread throughout the body by the time the primary site is detected. Surgery became more conservative: for example, a lumpectomy or partial mastectomy, which was followed by radiotherapy to the breast and/or with cytotoxic chemotherapy and hormone therapy used to treat the systemic disease.

There appears to be little difference in survival between local excision alone, local excision plus local radiotherapy, and modified

---

**Box 10.6** Staging of breast cancer—TNM definitions

**Primary tumor (T)**
- TX: Primary tumor cannot be assessed
- T0: No evidence of primary tumor
- Tis: Carcinoma in situ: DCIS or LCIS or Paget's disease of the nipple with no associated tumor[a]
- T1: Tumor 2 cm or less in greatest dimension
  —T1mic: Microinvasion, 0.1 cm or less in greatest dimension
  —T1a: Tumor more than 0.1 cm but not more than 0.5 cm in greatest dimension
  —T1b: Tumor more than 0.5 cm but not more than 1.0 cm in greatest dimension
  —T1c: Tumor more than 1 cm but not more than 2 cm in greatest dimension
- T2: Tumor more than 2 cm but not more than 5 cm in greatest dimension
- T3: Tumor more than 5 cm in greatest dimension
- T4: Tumor has spread to chest wall or to skin, only as described below
  —T4a: Direct extension to chest wall tissue (not including pectoralis muscle)
  —T4b: Direct extension to skin, showing edema (peau d'orange), ulceration, or skin nodules
  —T4c: Combined T4a and T4b
  —T4d: Inflammatory carcinoma

**Clinical regional lymph node involvement (N) (on *same* side as breast cancer)**
- NX: Node status cannot be assessed
- N0: No regional lymph node metastasis
- N1: Metastasis to moveable, ipsilateral axillary lymph nodes
- N2: Metastases in ipsilateral axillary lymph nodes fixed or matted, or in clinically apparent[b] ipsilateral internal mammary nodes with negative axillary nodes
  —N2a: Metastasis in ipsilateral axillary lymph nodes fixed to one another (matted) or to other structures
  —N2b: Metastasis only in clinically apparent[b] ipsilateral internal mammary nodes in the absence of clinically evident axillary lymph node metastasis
- N3: Metastasis in ipsilateral infraclavicular lymph nodes with or without axillary lymph node involvement, or in clinically apparent[b] ipsilateral internal mammary lymph node(s) and in the presence of clinically evident axillary lymph node metastasis; or metastasis in supraclavicular lymph node(s) with or without axillary or internal mammary lymph node involvement
  —N3a: Metastasis in ipsilateral infraclavicular lymph node(s)
  —N3b: Metastasis in ipsilateral internal mammary lymph node(s) and axillary lymph node(s)
  —N3c: Metastasis in ipsilateral supraclavicular lymph node(s)

**Distant metastasis (M)**
- MX: Presence of distant metastasis cannot be assessed
- M0: No distant metastasis
- M1: Distant metastasis

---

[a] Paget's disease associated with a tumor is classified according to the size of the tumor.
[b] Clinically apparent is defined as detected by imaging studies (excluding lymphoscintigraphy), or by clinical examination, or grossly visible pathologically.

**Table 10.7** Breast cancer—stage groups

| Stage | Primary tumor | Regional node involvement | Distant metastasis |
|-------|---------------|---------------------------|--------------------|
| 0 | Tis | N0 | M0 |
| I | T1[a] | N0 | M0 |
| IIA | T0 | N1 | M0 |
| | T1[a] | N1 | M0 |
| | T2 | N0 | M0 |
| IIB | T2 | N1 | M0 |
| | T3 | N0 | M0 |
| IIIA | T0 | N2 | M0 |
| | T1[a] | N2 | M0 |
| | T2 | N2 | M0 |
| | T3 | N1 | M0 |
| | T3 | N2 | M0 |
| IIIB | T4 | N0 | M0 |
| | T4 | N1 | M0 |
| | T4 | N2 | M0 |
| IIIC | Any T | N3 | M0 |
| IV | Any T | Any N | M1 |

[a]T1 includes T1mic (see Box 10.6).

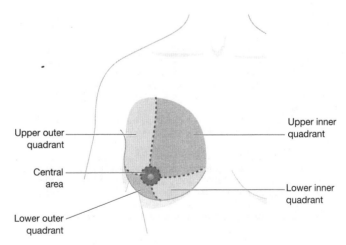

**Figure 10.6** Quadrants of the breast.

radical mastectomy; however, the more aggressive the treatment, the lower the chance of local recurrence. Local recurrence is associated with a worse survival rate but is probably an indicator of poor prognosis rather than being the cause of it. What ultimately

**Box 10.7** Pathological staging of lymph nodes for breast cancer—node status definitions

- pN0: Negative by histology (H&E) only; no additional examination for isolated tumor cells (ITC)
  —pN0(i−): H&E and IHC negative
  —pN0 (i+): H&E negative and IHC positive; no cell cluster bigger than 0.2 mm
  —pN0 (mol−): H&E and molecular findings negative
  —pN0 (mol+): H&E negative and molecular findings positive
- pN1: Metastases in 1–3 axillary nodes and/or in internal mammary nodes with microscopic disease detected by sentinel lymph node dissection but not clinically apparent[a]
  —pN1mi: Micrometastases >0.2 mm, none >2 mm
  —pN1a: Metastasis in 1–3 axillary lymph nodes
  —pN1b: Metastasis in internal mammary nodes, with microscopic disease detected by sentinel lymph node dissection but not clinically apparent[a]
  —pN1c: Metastasis in 1–3 axillary lymph nodes and in internal mammary nodes, with microscopic disease detected by sentinel lymph node dissection but not clinically apparent[a]
- pN2: Metastasis in 4–9 axillary lymph nodes, or in clinically apparent[b] internal mammary lymph nodes in the absence of axillary lymph node metastasis
  —pN2a: Metastasis in 4–9 axillary lymph nodes, at least one tumor deposit greater than 2 mm
  —pN2b: Metastasis in clinically apparent[b] internal mammary node(s) with negative axillary nodes
- pN3: Metastasis in 10 or more axillary lymph nodes, or in infraclavicular lymph nodes, or in clinically apparent[b] ipsilateral internal mammary lymph nodes in the presence of one or more positive axillary lymph nodes; or in more than 3 axillary lymph nodes with clinically negative microscopic metastasis in internal mammary lymph nodes; or in ipsilateral supraclavicular lymph nodes
  —pN3a: Metastasis in 10 or more axillary lymph nodes, with at least one tumor deposit larger than 2 mm, or metastasis to infraclavicular nodes
  —pN3b: Metastasis in clinically apparent[b] ipsilateral internal mammary nodes in association with one or more positive axillary lymph nodes; or in more than 3 axillary nodes and in internal mammary nodes with microscopic disease detected by sentinel lymph node dissection but not clinically apparent[a]
  —pN3c: Metastasis in ipsilateral supraclavicular lymph nodes

H&E, hematoxylin and eosin staining; IHC, immunohistochemical marker staining.
[a] Not clinically apparent is defined as not detected by imaging studies (excluding lymphoscintigraphy), or by clinical examination.
[b] Clinically apparent is defined as detected by imaging studies (excluding lymphoscintigraphy), or by clinical examination, or grossly visible pathologically.

**Table 10.8** NPI score related to need for chemotherapy

|  | NPI Score | | |
| --- | --- | --- | --- |
|  | <3.4 | 3.4–5.4 | 5.4 |
| Overall survival at 15 years | 80% | 42% | 13% |
| Need for chemotherapy | Doubtful | May benefit | Needed |

determines survival is the presence of micrometastases at presentation, which is the reason for systemic treatment. There is some evidence, however, that not all cases are systemic, which means some patients may be overtreated. Although mortality from breast cancer is decreasing, there is increased mortality from the side effects of treatment. It is therefore important that treatment be tailored to the individual patient rather than to breast cancer as a whole. In order to select the appropriate treatment for an individual patient, prognostic factors, such as the Nottingham prognostic index (NPI) and the Van Nuys prognostic index (VNPI), are being used. Factors taken into account include tumor size, grade, and axillary node involvement.

For the NPI, the score is worked out according to the following formula:

$$NPI = 0.2 \times (\text{pathological tumor size (cm)} + \text{histological grade} + \text{axillary nodes})$$

The resulting groupings range from excellent to poor prognosis. These figures can also be used to determine whether the patient may benefit from chemotherapy (see Table 10.8).

The VNPI is used for DCIS in order to decide which management option may be best for an individual patient. It combines tumor size, surgical margin, and pathological nuclear classification to create a score. These three parameters are significant predictors of local recurrence. The score is worked out according to the following formula:

$$VNPI = (\text{tumor size} \times 0.749) + (\text{pathological nuclear points} \times 0.869) + (\text{margin} \times 0.864)$$

Table 10.9 shows the VNPI in relation to treatment options.

Using a prognostic index, different groups of patients can be identified. The good prognostic groups have a survival similar to those of age-matched controls without breast cancer and therefore

**Table 10.9** VNPI related to treatment options

|  | VNPI Score | | |
| --- | --- | --- | --- |
|  | 3 or 4 | 5–7 | 8 or 9 |
| Treatment option | Conservative breast surgery | Conservative breast surgery plus radiotherapy | Mastectomy |

are unlikely to benefit from aggressive forms of treatment following surgery. This is the group that is possibly overtreated. The poor prognostic group, on the other hand, benefits from intensive systemic treatment.

Estrogen receptor status is also an indicator of prognosis, irrespective of the stage of the disease. Those who are estrogen receptor-positive (ER+) have a longer disease-free and overall survival than ER-negative patients, who have a higher recurrence rate along with lower overall survival. Around 60% of ER+ patients will respond to hormone therapy. *Tamoxifen*, until recently, was the treatment of choice, with patients given treatment for life or until recurrence. Studies in the USA have shown that maximum benefit is at 5 years. ER+ patients benefit more from this type of treatment than ER– patients and may also benefit from chemotherapy in addition to tamoxifen.

*Aromatase inhibitors* represent a new development in the area of hormone therapy. These appear to be better tolerated than tamoxifen and show a reduced rate of contralateral breast cancer compared with tamoxifen. Another benefit of aromatase inhibitors is that they do not induce endometrial hyperplasia as tamoxifen does, and therefore they do not increase the risk of endometrial carcinoma. However, they do not protect against osteoporosis, which is a benefit of tamoxifen; therefore, other forms of treatment for osteoporosis may be necessary. Overall, the prognosis of breast cancer is improving, but it is difficult to accurately define prognosis, as it combines so many different factors.

## SELF-ASSESSMENT QUESTIONS

Answer true or false to the following. Answers are on page 245.

1. The uterus consists of two parts.
2. The endometrium is under hormonal control.
3. Cervical cancer is mainly a disease of women over 40 years of age.
4. Cervical screening has increased the diagnosis of invasive carcinoma.
5. Human papilloma virus is the main etiologic factor for carcinoma of the cervix.
6. The majority of cervical carcinomas are adenocarcinomas.
7. A Wertheim's hysterectomy includes the removal of the upper third of the vagina.
8. The main etiologic factor for endometrial carcinoma is related to hormonal activity.
9. Postmenopausal bleeding is the classic presentation for endometrial carcinoma.
10. The majority of endometrial carcinomas are squamous cell carcinomas.
11. The ovaries have two functions.
12. Ovarian cancer kills more women than any other gynecologic malignancy.
13. Ovarian carcinoma occurs more in women with many children.
14. Teratoma of the ovary tends to be benign.
15. Ovarian tumors may grow very large before symptoms become obvious.
16. Breast size is related to the number of lobules.
17. Most breast lymph drains to the axillary nodes.
18. Breast cancer can be under hormonal influence.
19. Breast cancer mainly develops in the glandular tissue.
20. Breast cancer only spreads via the lymphatic system.

# 11

# The skin

The skin is the largest and most accessible organ of the body. Together with its accessory organs—hair, nails, sweat glands, and sebaceous glands, and the associated blood vessels, nerves, and lymphatic vessels—it is referred to as the integumentary system. The accessory organs allow the skin to carry out its functions of protecting underlying tissue, regulating temperature by excreting perspiration, preventing excessive loss of inorganic and organic materials, receiving stimuli from the environment, and synthesizing vitamin D.

The skin is continuous with the mucosa of the digestive, respiratory, urinary, and reproductive systems at their external openings and also with the mucosa around the eye. On average, an adult has a skin surface of around $19\,000\,cm^2$ with a thickness varying between 0.5 and 3 mm. The skin is thinner on the dorsal (back) surfaces than on the ventral (front) surfaces. The skin consists of two main parts: the epidermis and dermis (see Fig. 11.1).

The epidermis is non-vascular (contains no blood or lymphatic vessels) and consists of four or five layers of stratified epithelium (see Box 11.1). Cells formed from the continuous cell division of the basal layer of the epidermis gradually become more rounded and then flattened and keratinized (deposition of an insoluble protein called keratin) as they mature and rise to the surface layer. The time from cell production in the basal layer to the loss or shedding at the surface is normally 4 weeks, although in abnormal conditions such as psoriasis this can lessen to 7–10 days.

The dermis has two main regions: papillary and reticular. The papillary region comprises the upper 20% of the dermis and has

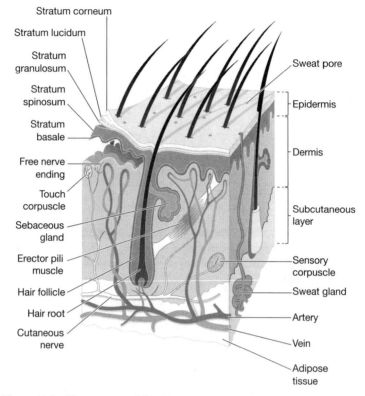

**Figure 11.1** The structure of the skin.

---

**Box 11.1** Layers of the epidermis

- *Stratum corneum*: 20–30 layers of flattened cells containing keratin; cells have no nuclei. This layer is continuously shed and replaced from the underlying layers. It forms a barrier to light, heat, water, chemicals, and bacteria
- *Stratum lucidium*: 3–5 rows of closely packed, clear, flat cells with traces of flattened nuclei; more pronounced in thicker areas of the skin such as the palms of the hands and soles of the feet; this layer is absent in hairy skin
- *Stratum granulosum*: 3–5 layers of flattening cells in which keratin is formed. Nuclear degeneration seen in this layer denotes dying cells; the keratinized cells release lipids that repel water
- *Stratum spinosum* (prickle cell layer): 8–10 rows of polygonal cells. Melanin is taken in from the nearby melanocytes
- *Stratum germinativum* (basal cell layer): the deepest layer; a single layer of columnar epithelium attached to a basement membrane; capable of continuous cell division, and containing melanocytes

finger-like projections called dermal papillae. It attaches the dermis to the epidermis and contains the capillaries carrying nutrients to the epidermis. Also within this layer are the sensory nerve endings for touch, pain, and temperature (see Fig. 11.1). The reticular region contains more dense, irregular connective tissue and also contains the sebaceous and sweat glands, fat and hair follicles. The dermis or dermal layer provides the elasticity of the skin. Under the dermis is a subcutaneous layer of adipose (fatty) tissue, the amount of which varies from person to person.

Skin color is determined by the amount of the pigment melanin in the epidermal cells. Everyone has the same number of melanocytes, but differing amounts of pigment produce a range of skin colors throughout the world. Freckles are caused by patches of melanocytes; albinism is the result of having no pigment; and vitiligo is an autoimmune condition in which there is a loss of melanocytes, causing white patches. In white skin, melanin is present in the basal, spinosum, and granulosum layers; in darker skin it is present in all layers. When exposed to ultraviolet radiation such as that from the sun, the amount and darkness of the pigment increases, producing tanning, which gives further protection against radiation. Blood vessels in the dermis also account for some coloration, such as blushing. Carotene present in the corneum and fatty areas of the dermis along with melanin gives yellow coloring to the skin.

## ONCOLOGY

Skin cancer is the most common of all malignancies worldwide but causes the fewest deaths. Incidence varies worldwide and is directly proportional to the intensity of sunlight, explaining why it is more common in Australia and South Africa than in Europe and North America. Mainly a disease of older age, skin cancer is rare under the age of 40. Malignant melanoma is more common in younger age groups than basal cell carcinoma (BCC) and squamous cell carcinoma (SCC). Overall, there is a slight male preponderance.

### Etiology

The main etiologic factor associated with skin cancer is sunlight. A high percentage of skin cancers arise on exposed parts of the body, more on outdoor workers than indoor workers. People with fair skin are more prone to skin cancer because of lack of the protective pigment melanin. Skin cancer is rare in darker-skinned populations, and when it does occur, there is equal incidence on exposed and unexposed parts of the body. Other causative factors include occupational carcinogens, X-rays, immune suppression, chronic ulcers, and scar tissue. Genetic factors have also been linked to skin cancer: for example, Gorlin's syndrome, an autosomal dominant condition which leads to multiple BCCs; and xeroderma pigmentosum, a rare autosomal recessive disorder that predisposes the individual to SCC.

## Types of skin cancer

The main skin cancer histologies to be considered are:

- basal cell carcinoma (BCC)
- squamous cell carcinoma (SCC)
- malignant melanoma.

## BCC and SCC

### BCC

The most common of the skin malignancies, BCC is also referred to as a *rodent ulcer*. Histologically, there is no evidence of maturation of the cells in the epidermis from the basal layer. The cells appear uniform with darkly stained nuclei and contain little cytoplasm. Their appearance can be nodular, pigmented, sclerosing, infiltrating, or ulcerative. Typically, BCC appears as a firm, pink papule with distinct raised edges and a slight depression or ulcerative center. They normally present as a non-inflammatory, painless 'spot' that becomes irritated and bleeds when scratched. BCCs are typically reported as a 'spot which does not heal'. Patients with a history of BCC should regularly check exposed skin, as multiple tumors are quite common. If left untreated, BCCs can invade locally, causing large areas of ulceration (hence the term rodent); they may destroy superficial cartilage and bone such as that around the nose and ears, but deep invasion is uncommon, as is metastatic spread, unless they break through the basement membrane below the basal layer.

---

**Box 11.2**  Staging of BCC and SCC of the skin—TNM definitions

**Primary tumor[a] (T)**
- TX: Primary tumor cannot be assessed
- T0: No evidence of primary tumor
- Tis: Carcinoma in situ
- T1: Tumor 2 cm or less in greatest dimension
- T2: Tumor more than 2 cm but not more than 5 cm in greatest dimension
- T3: Tumor more than 5 cm in greatest dimension
- T4: Tumor invades deep extradermal structures (i.e. cartilage, skeletal muscle, or bone)

**Regional lymph node involvement (N)**
- NX: Regional lymph nodes cannot be assessed
- N0: No regional lymph node metastasis
- N1: Regional lymph node metastasis

**Distant metastasis (M)**
- MX: Distant metastasis cannot be assessed
- M0: No distant metastasis
- M1: Distant metastasis

[a] Where there are multiple tumors, the one with the highest T category is classified and the number of separate tumors indicated, e.g. T2 (5)

---

## SCC

SCCs are less common than BCCs, even though they are associated with the same etiologic factors. Histologically, they typically appear as keratinizing squamous lesions in which the squamous cells penetrate the basement membrane below the basal layer and form clusters of cells in the subepithelial layer. Invasion through the basement membrane into the subepithelial layer increases the likelihood of local lymph node metastases, unlike BCCs, which tend not to penetrate this membrane. They typically appear as a crusted, scaly ulcer or an exophytic-type nodule that can be clinically difficult to distinguish from a BCC. Lesions arising at the mucocutaneous junctions tend to be more aggressive, as do those that appear in sites where the skin has been irradiated.

## Staging

Box 11.2 and Table 11.1 show the TNM definitions and stage groups for BCC and SCC.

**Table 11.1** BCC and SCC of the skin—stage groups

| Stage | Primary tumor | Regional node involvement | Distant metastasis |
|-------|---------------|---------------------------|--------------------|
| 0 | Tis | N0 | M0 |
| I | T1 | N0 | M0 |
| II | T2 | N0 | M0 |
| | T3 | N0 | M0 |
| III | T4 | N0 | M0 |
| | Any T | N1 | M0 |
| IV | Any T | Any N | M1 |

*Treatment*

Lesions should be diagnosed histologically before treatment is given. This includes a biopsy that may also be the only treatment for small lesions. There are various treatments available for BCCs and SCCs, including electrocautery, cryosurgery, topical chemotherapy, excisional surgery, and external beam radiotherapy. The choice of treatment depends on the site of the tumor, the cosmetic result of treatment, the availability of equipment, and patient preference. All are highly effective, with around a 90% cure rate. Radiotherapy is especially useful round the eye and nose, which are difficult surgical sites, for lesions such as the temple and forehead where there is less skin for surgical repair, and for large tumors that would require reconstructive surgery.

# Malignant melanoma

The incidence of malignant melanoma is doubling every 10 years. The main causative factor is sun exposure, in particular the amount of sunlight received, which correlates with distance from the equator. This applies for both exposed and unexposed parts of the body. Incidence varies worldwide, with Australia having an incidence four times that of the UK. The evidence incriminating sunlight includes the greater prevalence in outdoor workers, the higher incidence in fair-skinned people and younger people, the association with sunburn, and migration studies. Only 1% of the increase in incidence is thought to be connected with ozone depletion. Melanoma affects younger age groups more than do other skin cancers. It is twice as common in women than in men, with women having 50% on the legs and 15% on the trunk, whereas in men melanoma is less common on the legs, with 50% occurring on the trunk. Risk factors associated with malignant melanoma relate to the amount, or rather the lack, of melanin; therefore, there is a higher risk for those with fair hair and freckled skin. Other risk factors include a history of severe sunburn, a large number of moles, dysplastic nevi, and a family history not connected with sun exposure. Most organs of the body have been found at postmortem to be capable of harboring primary melanotic foci—for example, the larynx, esophagus, and bronchi. All contain clusters of melanocytes, but why the malignant change occurs is not known.

Malignant melanoma is divided into cellular subtypes, but these do not have independent prognostic or therapeutic significance. They include superficial spreading, nodular, lentigo maligna, acral lentiginous (palmar/plantar and subungual), and miscellaneous other cell types.

### Staging

Malignant melanoma can be staged by vertical thickness (Breslow's classification) and/or anatomic level of local invasion (Clark's levels), as well as TNM (see Box 11.3 and Table 11.2). The thickness of the malignant melanoma and the extent of local and distant spread are closely related to prognosis, and therefore it is important that the stage of disease be carefully evaluated before treatment is discussed.

There have been some changes to the staging of malignant melanoma to take into account advances from research and progress in staging techniques. These relate to the prognostic factors of ulceration of the primary and lymphatic spread and include five major changes:

- Tumor thickness has replaced Clark's level of invasion as this is a better predictor of survival.
- The primary tumor staging now includes whether ulceration is present or not.
- The number of lymph nodes in the N staging is now used rather than the size of the nodes involved.
- Clinical and pathological staging systems are now being used to include lymphatic mapping and the presence of micrometastatic disease in the lymph nodes.
- The M staging has been subdivided to include the anatomic site of the metastases and the level of serum lactate dehydrogenase (LDH).

**Box 11.3** Staging of malignant melanoma—definitions for TNM and Clark's classification

### Clark's level
- I: Lesions involving only the epidermis; not invasive
- II: Invasion of the papillary dermis, not reaching the papillary–reticular interface; no ulceration
- III: Invasion fills and expands papillary dermis, but does not penetrate reticular dermis; no ulceration
- IV: Invasion into reticular dermis but not subcutaneous tissue
- V: Invasion into subcutaneous tissue

### Primary tumor (T)
- TX: Primary tumor cannot be assessed
- T0: No evidence of primary tumor
- Tis: Melanoma in situ (atypical melanocytic hyperplasia, severe melanocytic dysplasia); not an invasive lesion
- T1: Tumor 1.0 mm or less thickness, with or without ulceration
  —T1a: Tumor 1.0 mm or less in thickness, without ulceration
  —T1b: Tumor 1.0 mm or less in thickness, with ulceration
- T2: Tumor more than 1.0 mm, but not more than 2.0 mm thickness, with or without ulceration
  —T2a: Tumor more than 1.0 mm, but not more than 2.0 mm thickness, without ulceration
  —T2b: Tumor more than 1.0 mm, but not more than 2.0 mm thickness, with ulceration
- T3: Tumor more than 2.0 mm but not more than 4 mm thickness, with or without ulceration
  —T3a: Tumor more than 2.0 mm but not more than 4 mm thickness, without ulceration
  —T3b: Tumor more than 2.0 mm but not more than 4 mm thickness, with ulceration
- T4: Tumor more than 4.0 mm thickness, with or without ulceration
  —T4a: Tumor more than 4.0 mm thickness, without ulceration
  —T4b: Tumor more than 4.0 mm thickness, with ulceration

### Regional lymph node involvement (N)
- NX: Regional lymph nodes cannot be assessed
- N0: No regional lymph node metastasis
- N1: Metastasis to one lymph node
  —N1a: Clinically occult (microscopic) metastasis in one node
  —N1b: Clinically apparent (macroscopic) metastasis in one node
- N2: Metastasis to 2 or 3 lymph nodes or intralymphatic regional metastasis, without nodal metastasis
  —N2a: Clinically occult (microscopic) metastasis in 2–3 nodes
  —N2b: Clinically apparent (macroscopic) metastasis in 2–3 nodes
  —N2c: In-transit metastasis or satellite(s), without lymph node metastasis
- N3: Metastasis to 4 or more regional lymph nodes, or matted lymph nodes, or in-transit metastasis or satellite(s) with metastatic lymph node(s)

### Distant metastasis (M)
- MX: Distant metastases cannot be assessed
- M0: No distant metastases
- M1a: Distant skin, subcutaneous, or lymph node metastases with normal serum LDH
- M1b: Lung metastasis with normal serum LDH
- M1c: All other visceral metastases with normal serum LDH or any distant metastases with elevated serum LDH

LDH, lactate dehydrogenase.

**Table 11.2** Malignant melanoma—stage groups

| Stage | Primary tumor | Regional node involvement | Distant metastasis |
|---|---|---|---|
| 0 | Tis | N0 | M0 |
| IA | T1a | N0 | M0 |
| IB | T1b | N0 | M0 |
| | T2a | N0 | M0 |
| IIA | T2b | N0 | M0 |
| | T3a | N0 | M0 |
| IIB | T3b | N0 | M0 |
| | T4a | N0 | M0 |
| IIC | T4b | N0 | M0 |
| III | Any T | N1 | M0 |
| | Any T | N2 | M0 |
| | Any T | N3 | M0 |
| IV | Any T | Any N | M1 |

Breslow' classification states that a tumor of thickness less than 1 mm poses a small risk of spread, whereas one 1.5 mm thick or more has a greater chance of spread.

### Diagnosis and treatment

Surgery is the treatment of choice for malignant melanoma, followed by chemotherapy. There is no oncological reason for not doing a biopsy, since this removes tumor for staging, prognosis, and treatment. A complete family history should be taken, and the whole body should be examined for lymphatic spread and liver/spleen involvement. A wide excision, which used to be the treatment of choice, cannot guarantee to the patient that the prognosis will be better. Although malignant melanoma spreads via the lymphatics, removing regional lymph nodes makes no difference to survival. Radiotherapy is not used except when surgery is not suitable. As many tumors are on the extremities, a high dose can be given without damage to internal structures, and radiation is also useful as palliation of secondary deposits in brain and bone.

### Prognosis

Prognosis is closely linked to the size and ulceration of the tumor, along with local and distant metastatic spread. Melanomas of thickness less than 1 mm have a 5-year survival of at least 90%, dropping to 40–50% if the lesion is over 4 mm in thickness.

## SELF-ASSESSMENT QUESTIONS

Answer true or false to the following. Answers are on page 245.

1. Hairy skin has the same number of epidermal layers as non-hairy skin.
2. The number of melanocytes gives skin its color.
3. The main etiologic factor for skin cancer is sunlight.
4. Tumors arising at the junction of the skin and mucosa tend to be more aggressive.
5. A rodent ulcer is another name for a squamous cell carcinoma.
6. Basal call carcinomas (BCCs) normally present as a non-inflammatory 'spot that does not heal'.
7. Multiple BCCs are uncommon.
8. BCCs do not commonly metastasize.
9. Squamous cell carcinomas (SCCs) are less common than BCCs.
10. SCCs do not penetrate the basement membrane.
11. Multiple BCCs and SCCs are staged according to the one with the highest T category.
12. All melanomas are malignant.
13. Malignant melanomas are more common nearer the equator.
14. Malignant melanomas affect younger age groups than other skin cancers.
15. Fair-haired people are at less risk of developing malignant melanoma.
16. The prognosis of malignant melanoma is dependent on cellular subtype.
17. The thickness of a malignant melanoma is related to the prognosis.
18. Surgery is the treatment of choice for malignant melanoma.
19. Wide surgical excision is related to a better prognosis.
20. Malignant melanomas spread via the lymphatics.

# Answers to self-assessment questions

## Chapter 1

| | | | | |
|---|---|---|---|---|
| 1. T | 2. F | 3. F | 4. F | 5. T |
| 6. F | 7. F | 8. T | 9. F | 10. T |
| 11. T | 12. T | 13. F | 14. T | 15. F |
| 16. F | 17. F | 18. T | 19. T | 20. F |

## Chapter 2

| | | | | |
|---|---|---|---|---|
| 1. F | 2. F | 3. T | 4. T | 5. T |
| 6. F | 7. F | 8. T | 9. T | 10. T |
| 11. F | 12. F | 13. F | 14. T | 15. T |
| 16. T | 17. F | 18. F | 19. T | 20. T |

## Chapter 3

| | | | | |
|---|---|---|---|---|
| 1. T | 2. F | 3. T | 4. F | 5. T |
| 6. F | 7. T | 8. F | 9. T | 10. T |
| 11. T | 12. T | 13. F | 14. T | 15. T |
| 16. F | 17. T | 18. T | 19. T | 20. F |

## Chapter 4

| | | | | |
|---|---|---|---|---|
| 1. T | 2. F | 3. T | 4. T | 5. F |
| 6. F | 7. F | 8. T | 9. F | 10. F |
| 11. T | 12. F | 13. T | 14. T | 15. F |
| 16. F | 17. T | 18. T | 19. F | 20. T |

## Chapter 5

| | | | | |
|---|---|---|---|---|
| 1. F | 2. T | 3. T | 4. T | 5. F |
| 6. T | 7. T | 8. F | 9. T | 10. F |
| 11. T | 12. F | 13. F | 14. T | 15. T |
| 16. T | 17. F | 18. T | 19. F | 20. T |

## Chapter 6

| | | | | |
|---|---|---|---|---|
| 1. F | 2. T | 3. T | 4. F | 5. F |
| 6. F | 7. T | 8. T | 9. T | 10. F |
| 11. T | 12. F | 13. F | 14. F | 15. T |
| 16. F | 17. T | 18. T | 19. T | 20. F |

## Chapter 7

| | | | | |
|---|---|---|---|---|
| 1. T | 2. F | 3. F | 4. T | 5. F |
| 6. T | 7. T | 8. T | 9. F | 10. F |
| 11. T | 12. T | 13. T | 14. F | 15. T |
| 16. T | 17. F | 18. T | 19. F | 20. T |

## Chapter 8

| | | | | |
|---|---|---|---|---|
| 1. T | 2. F | 3. T | 4. F | 5. T |
| 6. T | 7. F | 8. F | 9. T | 10. T |
| 11. F | 12. T | 13. F | 14. F | 15. F |
| 16. F | 17. T | 18. T | 19. F | 20. T |

## Chapter 9

| | | | | |
|---|---|---|---|---|
| 1. F | 2. T | 3. T | 4. F | 5. F |
| 6. T | 7. T | 8. T | 9. T | 10. T |
| 11. F | 12. T | 13. T | 14. T | 15. T |
| 16. T | 17. T | 18. F | 19. F | 20. T |

## Chapter 10

| | | | | |
|---|---|---|---|---|
| 1. F | 2. T | 3. F | 4. F | 5. T |
| 6. F | 7. T | 8. T | 9. T | 10. F |
| 11. T | 12. T | 13. F | 14. T | 15. T |
| 16. F | 17. T | 18. T | 19. T | 20. F |

## Chapter 11

| | | | | |
|---|---|---|---|---|
| 1. F | 2. F | 3. T | 4. T | 5. F |
| 6. T | 7. F | 8. T | 9. T | 10. F |
| 11. T | 12. F | 13. T | 14. T | 15. F |
| 16. F | 17. T | 18. T | 19. F | 20. T |

# Index

Larynx (*contd*)
  carcinoma
    prognosis 118
    stage groups *117*
    TNM definitions *116–17*
  oncology 115–18
Laser
  microsurgery 115
  surgery, cervical cancer 205
Leukemia 33
  acute
    lymphoblastic 43
    lymphocytic 43, 49
    myeloblastic 43
    myelocytic 46–7
    myeloid *38–9*
  chronic
    eosinophilic 45
    lymphocytic 49
    myeloid 45–6
    myelomonocytic 44
    neutrophilic 45
  lymphoid 43
  myeloid 43
Leukoplakia 129, 218
Leydig cells 174, 177
Li–Fraumeni syndrome 65
Lip cancer 131
  stage groups *131*
Lipids, solubility 4
Liver 147–9
  cancer
    stage groups *149*
    TNM definitions *149*
  lobes **148**
Loop electrosurgical excision
    procedure 205
Lumpectomy 225
Lungs 118–**119**
  cancer, cellular classification *120*
  non–small cell carcinoma 120
    stage groups *123*
    staging 121
    TNM definitions *122*
    treatment 121, 123
  oncology 119–23
  small cell carcinoma 120, 121
Lymph nodes 37, 40
  distribution **41**
  head and neck drainage **129**
  staging in breast cancer *220*
Lymphatic drainage, breast 213
Lymphatic nodules, aggregated
    40, 42
Lymphatic system 35, 37–42

Lymphoid cells, function 37
Lymphoid differentiation pathway
    35
Lymphoid neoplasms 35, *38–40*, 47
Lymphoma 35, 42, 47, 50–54
  intracerebral 86–7
  nasopharyngeal 103–4
  oncology 50
Lysodren 101

## M

M component 26
Malignancy, degree estimation 19
Mammography 215
Mast cell diseases *40*
Medulloblastoma 86–7
Meiosis 8–9
Melanin 236, 239
Melanoma
  malignant 238–41
    cellular subtypes 239
    Clark's classification 239, *240*
    prognosis 241
    stage groups *241*
    staging 239, *240–1*
    TNM definitions *240*
MEN syndrome 98, 102
Meninges 82, **83–4**
Menstruation 204
6-Mercaptopurine 49
Mesenchymal cells 10, 13
  differentiation pathways 57–**58**
Mesenchyme 9
Mesoderm 9, 57
Mesothelioma 124
Metaphase 8
Metastasis 17–18, 19
Methotrexate 48–9
Microglioma *79*
Microsurgery, laser 111
Mitomycin C 165
Mitosis 5, 7–8
  phases **6**
Mitotane 101
Mitotic index 20
Mitoxantrone 46
Molecule
  carrier, presence 4
  size 4
MOPP 52
Multiple Endocrine Neoplasia (MEN)
    syndrome 98, 102